BRIDGING Science *and* Spirit

The Genius of William A. Tiller's
Physics and the Promise of Information Medicine

NISHA J. MANEK, MD

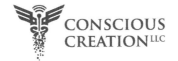

CONSCIOUS
CREATION LLC

PRAISE
FOR *BRIDGING SCIENCE AND SPIRIT*

❝*Experiencing Dr. Nisha Manek's presentations on the subject of integrative health, science, and consciousness is a true pleasure for our community of scholars and researchers at the California Institute for Human Science. Her work with Dr. Bill Tiller is forefront in the field of consciousness studies. Her book* Bridging Science and Spirit *coalesces the vision of these two maverick scientists and innovative thinkers. It takes us to the edge of current research on the limits, or lack thereof, of consciousness and the awesome potential of integrative healthcare beyond what was thought possible. I will enjoy using this text with CIHS graduate students to demonstrate these seminal issues and the interstices of Dr. Tiller's and Dr. Manek's work.*❞

—HOPE PHILLIPS UMANSKY, PhD
CEO and Academic Dean of the California Institute for Human Science

❝ *Human beings are by our very nature contemplative beings, endowed with a unique capacity to reflect and to intend. Dr. Manek reveals compelling new scientific evidence that human intention operates in the quantum field and that intention can impact the health and wellbeing of yourself and others. You will find* Bridging Science and Spirit *a godsend.* ❞

—JEFF GENUNG
President and Co-founder, Contemplative Life

The movement to merge modern science and thousands of years of mystical science—the known of transcendence through experience—has been slow. The father of the field of psychoenergetics, William A. Tiller, PhD, has been one of few experts leading this movement. His massive contribution to this movement is in need of greater public awareness. And with this in mind, Dr. Nisha Manek, the internationally recognized leader of integrative medicine, wrote Bridging Science and Spirit. *In the book, Dr. Manek summarizes two hundred hours of her personal meetings with Dr. Tiller. The book unravels not only core concepts of psychoenergetics but also Tiller's concept of 'Information Medicine is the way of the future.' I find the book style is very entertaining, easy to read, and most of all, soul awakening.*

– MIKHAIL KOGAN, MD

Medical Director, George Washington Center for Integrative Medicine, Associate Director, Geriatric Fellowship, George Washington University, and Founder and President, AIM Health Institute

Prepare yourself for an unrelenting encounter with deep awe and wonderment. Manek writes brilliantly. She takes the geek, mystic, and artist in us on a journey across familiar thresholds into Tiller's world of deep pivots, displacement of the known, and stunning entries into the unknown blossoming at the edge of our most profound concerns and wildest imagining. At the end of this read, you may find hefty walls of the known that framed your view are fallen, gone, no more. In their stead, you may feel and sense the impossible careening into the possible at the twinkling of an eye! And if you are like me, you'll realize you've lived to experience information with the power to incite metanoia within the human collective, enabling the evolution of our species to harmonize with nature and our origins.

Resplendent joy rushes in as you feel the silent landscape dormant within ripened onto an illumined path of radiance that informs and expresses wholly. Yowja! Yowsa! Yowsah! Yowza! 🙶

– **MYRA L. JACKSON**
Host of Gaiafield Radio, UN Harmony with Nature Expert,
and Sr. Advisor, Geoversity Foundation

BRIDGING SCIENCE AND SPIRIT:

The Genius of William A. Tiller's Physics and the Promise of Information Medicine

By Nisha J. Manek, MD

Illustrated by Dario Paniagua

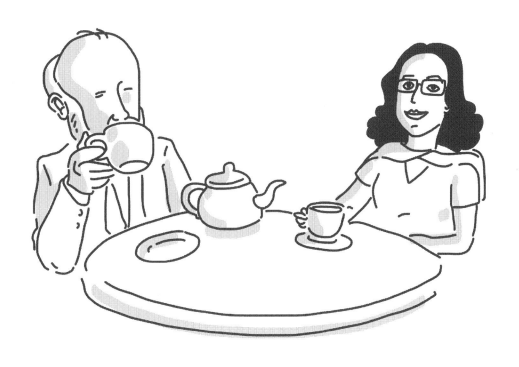

Bridging Science and Spirit: The Genius of William A. Tiller's Physics and the Promise of Information Medicine®

Information Medicine® is a trademark registered in the United States Patent and Trademark Office.

Book cover design and illustrations by Dario Paniagua (www.dariopaniagua.com)

Interior design by BookNook.biz

Editing & fact-checking by Eye Comb Editors (www.eyecombeditors.com)

Proofreading by Ann Aubrey Hanson (www.annaubrey.com)

Nisha Manek books are available for order through Amazon.com.

Visit my website: www.NishaManekMD.com
Follow me on Twitter: @nishamanekmd

Connect with me on Facebook:
www.facebook.com/Bridging-Science-and-Spirit

Printed in the United States of America
First printing: September 2019
Published by Conscious Creation LLC

Library of Congress Control Number: 2019905382

ISBN-13: paperback: 978-1-950559-00-8
ISBN-13: eBook: 978-1-950559-01-5
ISBN-13: hardback: 978-1-950559-02-2

Disclaimer: The contents of this book, such as text, graphics, images, and other material contained in the appendices ("Content") are for informational purposes only; the Content is not intended to be a substitute for professional medical advice, diagnosis, or treatment. The author does not give medical advice herein, and no doctor–patient relationship is offered or created. Always seek the guidance of your own doctor with questions you may have regarding your health or a medical condition before pursuing any kind of medical treatment. The author does not recommend, endorse, or make any representation about any tests, practices, procedures, treatments, services, opinions, health care providers, physicians, or medical institutions that may be mentioned or referenced herein. Never disregard the advice of a medical professional, or delay in seeking it because of something you have read in this book. If you choose to rely on any information provided in *Bridging Science and Spirit*, you do so solely at your own risk. Under no circumstances are the author or the Tiller Institute responsible for the claims of third-party websites or educational providers.

Dedicated to the memory of my father, Jayantilal Liladhar Manek, who saw the bridge long before everyone.

And to my teachers: David Ramon Hawkins, MD, PhD, and Vimalaji Thakar, two radiant pillars.

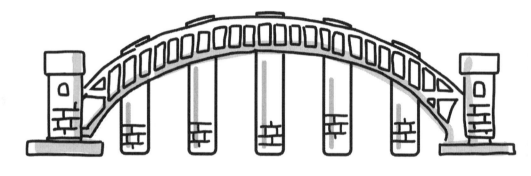

My long-term goal in the psychoenergetics area since 1970 has been to help build a reliable bridge of understanding for humans that seamlessly joins the foundations of traditional science on one end, extends through the domains of the psyche, emotion, and mind and is firmly planted in the bedrock of Spirit at the other end. And further, that this bridge is both strong enough and reliable enough that, eventually, normal folks and traditional scientists will joyfully walk across it.

—William A. Tiller

CONTENTS

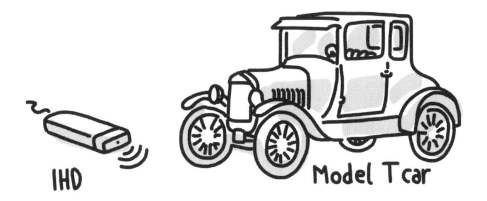

FOREWORD

In June 1972, I had the great privilege of meeting Dr. William Tiller at Stanford University during the first major US metaphysical and acupuncture meeting. There I was also introduced to Felix Mann, a British physician who practiced acupuncture in the heart of London; Gladys and Bill McGarey, who introduced me to Edgar Cayce's work; and Olga Worrall, the most-studied spiritual healer in history. Bill discussed, among other things, the Bonghan acupuncture channels and, even more, was able to discuss complex physics concepts in understandable terms. Indeed, he is far more comprehensible to the layman in his accessible lectures than he is in his scientific articles. Since that time, I have had many opportunities to talk with him about a wide variety of subjects, ranging from intention to multidimensional universes. From a scientific point of view, his work with intentionally imprinted simple electric-circuit devices that can enhance liver enzymes and shorten the lifecycle of fruit flies is revolutionary. Bill's protocol to increase well-being in people by broadcasting information via his imprinted device is a remarkable potential advancement in modern therapeutics.

Perhaps his concept of vector field or empty space helped me most of all. Vector energy fills *all* empty space in the universe. Although the magnitude of this energy cannot be measured directly, according to Bill, the empty space in a single hydrogen atom contains enough energy to boil the oceans if it is properly focused! To me, this means vector energy is the physical manifestation of the power of God.

Indeed, intention and programming of devices to influence people, time, and space are all aspects of spirituality, of our intimate experience of the Divine. I know of no physicist who lives more intimately in God or the Divine world. His Virgo personality is a perfect blend of organized science and spirituality.

I expect *Bridging Science and Spirit* to become popular in the pantheon of books exploring consciousness. It will inform, educate, and even entertain readers.

—C. NORMAN SHEALY, MD, PhD
Author of *Conversations with G:
A Physician's Encounter with Heaven*

PREFACE

There are many books that study consciousness and intention in great detail. This book is not one of them. Rather, *Bridging Science and Spirit* looks at the major themes of Professor William A. Tiller's physics, of Tillerian physics. Each major theme is a pillar, and successive pillars are connected into a bridge that allows us to cross between today's science at one end and Spirit at the other end. Each pillar is constructed with essays that form individual "bricks." Essays may seem an idiosyncratic choice for communicating the profound science of Tillerian physics. By necessity, dealing with broad subjects in a few words is, to some extent, a problem of design and engineering. So I had to be an engineer and select which of Tiller's key ideas I would write about; it was a value judgment on my part. In this way, the great span between science and Spirit could be bridged. Where before there was nothing, now there is something. There are no "proofs" in this book, but instead a glimpse into how one scientist sees God's work in us and in nature.

Each essay opens with a Tiller quotation. His words are unchanged, with minor adjustments inserted in brackets. The bricks (essays) construct and support the main pillar theme from related aspects, just as a bridge has a foundation with supporting cables. Unless indicated otherwise, all Tiller quotations in the book are from my in-person conversations with him. Most are Tiller sayings familiar to those who know him well.

At my first dinner meeting with Tiller, my copy of his book

Psychoenergetic Science: The Second Copernican Scale Revolution in hand, I suggested to him: "You need to have visuals and diagrams to communicate your ideas."[1]

Tiller looked thoughtful and replied: "That's your job." I took on that task, and Dario Paniagua transformed my basic sketches into illustrations. Illustration is about making communication easy, clear, and fun for the reader. Each essay has an illustration to visually describe the core idea. You may wish to keep a copy of *Psychoenergetic Science* as a go-to book while reading *Bridging Science and Spirit,* in which I present my independent scholarship.

As an author, I took creative license in reconstructing some well-known events in the history of science. The fundamental facts are true.

Initially, the first pillar may seem to have nothing to do with consciousness. This pillar centers on Truth and revolutions. It gives you a grasp of scientific history, the modern scientific path, and a perspective on some of the most pressing issues in modern medicine. We meet Nicolaus Copernicus and René Descartes and understand Tiller's core idea of subtle energies and psychoenergetics. Its structure concludes with the momentous discovery of twenty-first century physics: the Higgs boson.

In the second pillar, we will see that consciousness is not readily measurable in the way we might expect, that is, according to the methods of brain science. Instead, we will ask what consciousness *does.* This may sound technical, but in the quest to construct a useful bridge it is necessary to keep an engineering perspective and ask: "Will this structure hold for all time?"

The third pillar explores the mighty second law of thermodynamics and the new "hot" idea of dissipative systems. We will meet superstars like Ludwig Boltzmann, Jeremy England of the Massachusetts

Institute of Technology, and Claude Shannon, father of communication theory. This pillar's structure concludes with a practical look at how physics helps you choose the right nutritional diet.

In the fourth pillar, we dive right into the target experiments. The results are nothing short of stunning: Science is turned inside out and upside down.

In the bridge's fifth pillar, another giant of science makes an appearance: Paul Dirac. He is a key character in our bridge building, while others, like Albert Einstein, are here mere bit players. We discover a major principle of nature: the underlying structure of space itself and nature's symmetries. The presence of additional dimensions is probably the least objectionable feature of Tillerian physics; physicists have long wondered why space has three dimensions and time only one. Yet can space really have extra dimensions? It seems vague and mystical. You will learn the answer. The fifth pillar concludes with a thought experiment exploring the popular term "zero-point energy." For readers eager to get to this brick, you can skip ahead to essay 38.

In the sixth pillar, I address medicine—my thing—and showcase data from Information Medicine that can profoundly shape the way we approach disease and health and personalized medicine.

This leads to our final pillar, number seven: Spirit. It is as though, to anchor the bridge in the bedrock of Spirit, the Buddha himself extended a helping hand and gave an astounding confirmation of the Tillerian physics model.

So, visualize, expand your imagination, and have fun!

Nisha J. Manek

Yorba Linda, California

INTRODUCTION

By profession, I am a medical doctor. As a rheumatologist, I spent twelve years as a faculty member in a major academic hospital system. I have always been drawn to spirituality in its broadest sense, and most of my personal studies are in this area. I am a dedicated "seeker" and I value being at the center of something integral and critical. There are answers, and I am going to find them in this lifetime.

One day, I read Professor William Tiller's paper on consciousness with the formidable title "Expanding the Thermodynamic Perspective for Materials in an SU(2) Electromagnetic (EM) Gauge Symmetry State Space: Part I, A Duplex Space Model with Applications to Homeopathy."[2] I didn't know it at the time, but I was holding a paper about an astonishing scientific idea.

In retrospect, I now see that nothing was accidental about my stumbling into the world of psychoenergetic science and the relationship between intention and medicine. I read Tiller's paper thoroughly. Two things stood out. First, I didn't have a clue what the paper was about, and second, I knew in my bones that I had been handed a gift. Unconsciously, I perceived what Tiller was writing about—it made my heart race for no apparent reason. Consciously, thanks to my own resistance, I grasped every ninth word, if I was lucky. The paper's style was abstruse, even incomprehensible, with pages of equations and factors I did not recognize let alone comprehend, but its message set off a firestorm of inquiry in my mind that persists to this day. That was more than ten years ago.

Throughout my medical career, I always felt there was more than the cause-and-effect way we managed diseases. Patient outcomes regularly defied all the carefully constructed rules of medicine. The vague inner sense that there was more to healing than administering drugs remained. As a recipient of the Bravewell scholarship, I completed my associate fellowship diploma in integrative medicine from the University of Arizona in 2006. Although this opened a more holistic perspective for me, and I combined integrative and conventional care for arthritis disorders, science and spirituality still seemed disconnected and were mainly treated as separate in the clinic and hospital setting.

In my quest to find Truth, I recognized in Tiller someone like a sage. I checked the validity of my recognition in every way that I could and proved his genuineness to my complete satisfaction. "Checking him out" included examining his exceptional scientific pedigree. In this work of verification, sometimes the universe sends us an unexpected gift. While attending an integrative medicine conference in Washington, DC, I met the late Rustum Roy, professor at Pennsylvania State University and a leader in materials research. Roy, who knew about Tiller's work, told me: "His science is powerful."

I set my intention to meet Tiller and ask questions about the first paper of his I had read and its conclusions, which, frankly, escaped me, despite multiple readings. I sent him several emails and received . . . nothing. Then suddenly, out of the blue came a message from his associate, Dr. Walter Dibble. I hung on to every word in that singular email: "Bill says read his book *Psychoenergetic Science.*"

Finally, in 2009, while I was presenting talks in Scottsdale, Arizona, I left a message at his labs in Payson, Arizona. He accepted my invitation for a dinner meeting. I was there because of what I knew (or thought I knew) about the human biofield. But the degree to which I understood what he was saying mattered less than the impression he made. I was overwhelmed that someone of his stature would choose to spend his time discussing science with me. Over apple pie and French fries, he was generous, kind, attentive, and magnanimous.

In the course of that first meeting, I mentioned my study of *A Course in Miracles*. He and his wife, Jean, had been given a copy of the earliest draft of *A Course in Miracles* by none other than the scribe Helen Schucman, who visited their home at Stanford sometime in the mid-1970s. He said: "We both read and liked the course. The material [of the course] was very familiar to us. It is how we lived every day."

I was astounded. Here was a giant of a scientist who was also a giant in spirituality. It would have been no small gesture for fellow scientist Helen Schucman to come to Palo Alto and meet with the Tillers. For me, this was pivotal. I felt I had found my mentor. He autographed my copy of *Psychoenergetic Science,* "Much Love. Bill Tiller."

Teachers or gurus are people we meet along the way who have more wisdom than we do and, to our surprise, offer to share what they know. Except, he wasn't interested in mentoring any doctor. Luckily, a few months later, I received what I consider a most important phone call from Dr. Tiller. He explained that after thinking things through, he felt that maybe my role was to communicate to my medical colleagues the potential of Information Medicine. He also carefully and thoroughly cautioned me that he had no funds for my studies. No matter. I was in.

His second request to me revealed something of Tiller's depth. "You must meditate daily." Institutes and companies do not normally require their prospective hires to meditate, and it is certainly not a question asked on medical school applications! The importance he placed on inner development was, for me, both unexpected and thrilling.

In the dead of winter, I packed up my apartment in Rochester, Minnesota, got into my Jeep, and headed for Scottsdale, Arizona, driving furiously as an ice storm approached behind me. My idea was to study physics—thermodynamics, to be precise—with a clear end date of six months. I arrived in Scottsdale to commence my somewhat ill-defined duties as physics student or something or other. I would live in a short-term rental apartment in Scottsdale with an air mattress for a bed, a collection of physics books, and no external distractions. My apartment was three miles from the Tiller home. I went to work.

In early January 2011, as friends and colleagues celebrated the new year in the freezing Minnesota winter, I began weekly Thursday meetings with Bill Tiller in his sunny living room. An original oil painting by Ingo Swann—the father of remote viewing and a personal friend of the Tillers, hung on the wall, with its burst of blues and yellows over a horizon, like a silent, ever-present muse and guide to our discussions.

There was no formal curriculum, and like an intrepid traveler I decided what I wanted to explore during our two hours. Can a physician have anything in common with a physicist? We settled upon the study of "Information Medicine," which pleased us both. Within a couple of weeks, Tiller was driving the three miles to my sparse apartment every Thursday, and at precisely 9 a.m. we would begin our dialogue. I carefully balanced a flip camera on a thick stack of physics texts to record Tiller as he spoke, so that I could be present rather than trying to write everything down. After precisely two hours, Tiller would put his brown hat back on and, with twinkling eyes, say: "See you next week, kiddo!"

I have since spent three years and more than ninety Thursday meetings with Tiller. He is a splendid teacher. He loves questions and deep thought, and he has no snobbery about my lack of knowledge or my misinformation about physics. Instead, he seemed to like that there was this persistent and largely ignorant person who nevertheless loved to explore questions about what makes humans so darn special. Tiller treated me like a fellow scientist—nothing less, nothing more, which meant he treated me with respect.

When I look back on our meetings, I see them as one long conversation. In a way, that conversation continues as I sort through his vast archive of writings and white papers. Our discussions were lively, covering varied subjects, not just physics and medicine. In those two hours, we talked about meditation, contemplation, the latest science discoveries (such as the Higgs boson), and even new books on Amazon. What I discovered was that his every sentence had wrapped inside it, like a package, many concepts. It was up to me to unpack the concepts and produce my own picture, like a painting. "We are like artists," he would say. That way, I came to "own" the information and brought my unique voice to it. As you read, you will notice some technical stuff, simplified for general comprehension and due to my own understanding, which I am offering in its own maturation or lack thereof.

When I told people what I was doing in Scottsdale—not clinical medicine but a self-funded sabbatical in physics, they often shook their heads, as in, "You are crazy!" They were astonished. Although it appears that my life is "leisurely," it is no extended vacation. My life is a choice like any other, with its advantages and disadvantages. I sacrificed some things (like a steady job and income, security, and a sense of belonging among professional circles) for other things (like freedom to think and the chance to discover more about nature, human potential, and new paradigms in medicine). I feel honored and privileged to have made this choice.

My initial question to Tiller centered on the energy systems of the human body. But Tiller went much further than my question about biofields and shook the very foundations of all my beliefs, particularly those about the role of thermodynamic laws in doctor–patient interactions. Little did I know that I was going to engage in a long struggle between what we think and say there is and what might actually be. Little by little, materialism gave way to the Truth that reality isn't what I insist it is.

In the process of scientific discovery, when a new idea occurs to a scientist, it does not emerge in its final polished form. It is often confused and muddled, and it may take years, sometimes decades, before its consequences have been sufficiently thought out to put together an orderly presentation, as for example in Tiller's books *Conscious Acts of Creation* and *Some Science Adventures with Real Magic*. Tiller's astonishing take on solving the "hard problem" of consciousness is grounded in understanding reality beyond spacetime (the concepts of time and three-dimensional space regarded as fused in a four-dimensional continuum).[3] He does magic with a science protocol to test his intention and put a number to it, that is, quantify intention mathematically. He links what lies beyond spacetime to the here and now.

According to Tiller in his conversations with me, it happened like this:

"I went to Oxford University in 1973 for a yearlong postdoctoral study and to write a book on crystallography. But I just could not get my mind off the crazy stuff like remote viewing or how people could affect reality from a far distance. How could this weird stuff coexist with what I was studying every day at Stanford? I realized we need data. Good data. So, in my mind I held the question, like a brick in my hand, of how humans can do extraordinary things. What kind of physics is required? After daily meditations on this question, six months into my time at Oxford, I realized that there was no one else to do it. It had to be me."

Upon returning to California, Tiller created the conditions to enable him to pursue his research. Leaving his department chair position and advisory board memberships, he made time. He got to know his own "thought current" and augmented his intention, building a bridge within. He forayed into himself, and the intention research protocol gradually emerged. Throughout the 1980s and 1990s, while teaching materials science and engineering at Stanford University, Tiller drew inspiration from his outer world of hard science and inner work of daily readings of spiritual classics like the *Bhagavad Gita,* with a copy always on hand in his briefcase. His principle hypothesis was that directed human intention "in here" can change physical reality "out there" in a measurable way.

Few have heard of Tiller's book *Psychoenergetic Science.* There are various reasons for this unawareness. Two of them are obvious: language and subject matter. The term "psychoenergetic" is not easily understood. It describes links between the human psyche and energy. The subject of energy seems obvious, yet in the physical sciences, turn to any physics or chemistry text and look for a definition of "energy." You quickly find there is no precise definition of "energy." For the moment, I too am going to leave the subject of energy and let the bridge lead us to how Tiller represents it.

In his work, Tiller observed conventional and time-honored canons of the laboratory, aided by the current repertoire of instrumentation, Faraday shielding, and living systems. It was a perfectly regular and routine piece of scientific work, like the study of communication among birds, the luminescence of fireflies, how our muscles move, or any other emergent observations about nature. He set up four protocols to seek the answers to the question: Can human intention affect materials? And if so, how does this happen?

Inquiring into his physics, I came to feel that if I could discover where Tiller got his power—this power I didn't understand—if I could explain it, as Pulitzer prize-winning historian and biographer Robert Caro said of his own work, I would be adding something to the knowledge people ought to have about the power of intention. Not the kinds of things you read in books, but about the full real-world existence of power, about how power works in nature, and how it truly works in your life and around you.

Alongside Tiller was his wife, Jean "Jeannie." After they wed, Jeannie made it her business to create a cocoon in which her husband could think and write without worrying about the responsibilities of their home. Tiller helped establish many well-known institutes—Institute of Noetic Sciences (IONS), the Institute of HeartMath, the California Institute for Human Science, and more, while Jeannie took care of their two young children. She was an integral part of the team, a scientist in her own way, and her insights would lead to "aha" moments and forward momentum in some of Tiller's research. She stated that both she and Tiller have a daily meditation practice, which they have done for more than fifty years.

After he retired from Stanford University in 2000, the Tillers moved to Payson, Arizona. Within just a year or two, this firebrand physicist had constructed a whole new lab under the shade of pine trees. Some of our Thursday meetings were in the labs, now closed at the time of this writing. I would drive on Arizona highway 87, past the sleepy outpost that is Rye, to Payson at an ear-popping 4,800 feet above sea level. The Tiller compound was tucked away at the end of a cul-de-sac. There was nothing to tell passersby that there was anything outside of the ordinary inside the wide-open white iron gates. No name-board. No institute. No self-importance. Nothing grand.

Once inside the Tillers' Payson home, I might have made a parachute jump into another world far from the deserts and saguaro cacti of Arizona. There was magic in the very air. The lab space overflowed and spilled with monitors, Faraday cages, thermometers, computers, books, and papers, whose busyness camouflaged a deeper, more profound reality. The clue to me was the *feeling* of being in that Tiller lab: I would come away feeling a sense of well-being, like after sleeping all night and waking refreshed. Rejuvenated. I looked forward to the Thursdays we met at his Payson labs.

Tiller often talks about "the bridge of understanding." The main emphasis is on the general unifying principles that emerge from the great mass of detailed observations. A bridge does not "solve" problems or "explain" mysteries; a bridge merely helps us to locate them, identify them, and get across to the other side of greater understanding and coherence. In his imagination, a bridge is an edifice constructed to hold the weight of evidence together, with the invisible wonder of faith acting as cables and his inner vision as the structure's towers. This all rests on a hidden foundation buried deep inside. You can't see what underlies the structure, but it's there and everything else depends on the strength of this inner structure.

A bridge had to be built to benefit mankind, to unify two great and complementary pathways to Truth: science, and Spirituality. Tiller had to gather the necessary materials and engineer the whole thing. It takes time and courage to make bricks in the fire of experiment and data. And finally, we now have something arching over a chasm that previously looked untraversable.

Tiller belongs to the school of life: know life's limits, see its potential; see and analyze your own potential, build on what you have, and create. And be brave. Everything else is boring and won't work. Best of all, Tiller offers advice—not all of it based on decades of theoretical physics or conducting lab experiments, on the big eternal question: How should we live?

To NISHA:

WISHING YOU GREAT
AND ABUNDANT JOY
AS YOU CONTINUE TO EMBRACE
THE UNFOLDING ADVENTURE!

MUCH LOVE

Bill Tiller

A bridge is a place that is no place

at all, that is in itself *between*:

you belong, quite simply, to the bridge.

And then you keep walking

and reach the other side.

—Erica Wagner

in *Chief Engineer. Washington Roebling. The Man Who Built the Brooklyn Bridge.*[4]

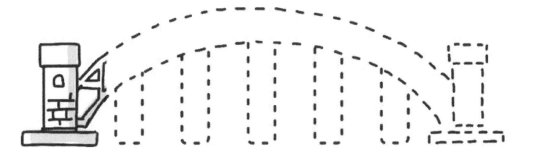

BRIDGE PILLAR 1:
Of Truth and Revolutions—Mankind Is Set Spinning and the Birth of the Miraculous Science

Bless the LORD, O my soul.
Who layeth the beams of his chambers in the waters:
who maketh the clouds his chariot: who walketh upon
the wings of the wind: Who laid the foundations of the earth,
that it should not be removed for ever
–PSALM 104:1, 3, 5

Of all discoveries and opinions, none may have exerted a greater
effect on the human spirit than the doctrine of Copernicus.
The world had scarcely become known as round and complete in
itself when it was asked to waive the tremendous privilege of being
the center of the universe. Never, perhaps, was a greater demand
made on mankind—for by this admission so many things vanished
in mist and smoke! What became of Eden, our world of innocence,
piety and poetry; the testimony of the senses; the conviction
of a poetic-religious faith? No wonder his contemporaries
did not wish to let all this go and offered every possible resistance

to a doctrine which in its converts authorized and demanded
a freedom of view and greatness of thought so far unknown,
indeed not even dreamed of.

—JOHANN WOLFGANG VON GOETHE in *Copernicus' Secret*[5]

[1]
"Copernicus set off a revolution in science."
When Heaven and Earth Moved

We hear about the next big revolution in science almost daily, whether it be artificial intelligence, gravitational waves, space travel for the ordinary man, or the possibility of humanity's new abode on Mars. We are like a family looking through travel brochures.[6] Years down the road, the next big thing takes over, and today's news fades into the dust of time and memory.

Tiller wastes no words with the title of his book, *Psychoenergetic Science: The Second Copernican-Scale Revolution.*[7] It is helpful to consider the significance of the word "revolution." What does it mean that science is revolutionary? Who decides what is revolutionary in the first place? What sets that science apart?

If you want to know how science works, there is a great advantage in actively working as a scientist, trying to tease out the structure of nature from among the ambiguities of observations made at the cutting edge of a field. A complementary approach is to examine some historical cases in depth, because the passage of time affords a helpful perspective.[8] Tiller appropriates Nicolaus Copernicus's science as the first revolution.

Let's journey back to 1512 in Varmia, Northern Poland. Not far from the brackish waters of the Vistula Lagoon stands Frauenburg Cathedral (known today as Frombork). Inside the dim light of Frauenburg Cathedral's entryway, we imagine the solitary figure of Copernicus, his head bowed reverently toward the triptych of the Virgin Mary. As the sun sets, he ascends the circular stone steps as he has often done before, to implore the night sky. If he is lucky, it will be cloudless without mists rolling in from the nearby waters of the Vistula. Training his eye through a thin metal tube—it was nearly a hundred years before the invention of the telescope—Copernicus scans the heavens, paying particular attention to the red-hued planet. Over many weeks, he has surveyed its march across the skies on an easterly course, its trajectory slowing down until it almost seems to waver and stop briefly. Then the planet reverses its direction and has gradually moved backward in a loop-the-loop toward the west, as though an unseen hand is beckoning it. Why did Mars behave so peculiarly?

Back in his chamber, Copernicus placed his quill on Earth. Using the accepted Claudius Ptolemy's geocentric cosmology, he set Mars swinging around Earth—the presumed fixed center of the universe, with a second circle, called an "epicycle," riding on the first one. Calculations using the combined circles of Ptolemy's arrangement provided Copernicus with an approximate solution for Mars's changing positions in the sky.[9] But this was not acceptable to him. What he must have done, to account for what he observed, was change the way the model worked.

Copernicus inked his quill and assuredly placed it on the *Sun* as the still point and set *both* Earth and Mars orbiting. In this heliocentric cosmology, Earth, being closer to the Sun, moves faster than the red planet. At times, Earth overtakes and passes Mars as both orbit the Sun. At those times, Mars appears to make a backward loop in the sky for a few months, in a direction contrary to its normal movement, called "retrograde." Now if Mars is retrograde, then that means one thing: Earth must not be standing still at a geocentric point (center of the Universe), as everyone believed. Instead, it and the other planets must revolve around the Sun.

As Copernicus studied his calculations by candlelight, the wick's tip, nearly at the bottom of the wax column, abruptly flared as though in confirmation, the large flame casting a golden glow on his earnest face and reflected in his dark eyes. He had deciphered the solar system![10] With heliocentrism, the entire entourage of planets arrange themselves so that the planet with the shortest orbital period, Mercury, orbits closest to the Sun, and Mars as well as the rest, such as the sluggish Saturn, fall in order proportionately. It also explained the mystery in Ptolemic astronomy. Mars, Jupiter, and Saturn periodically stop their eastward progress in the heavens and move westward in retrograde orbits. Copernicus's cosmos *required* retrograde motion, while Ptolemy's merely *allowed* for it. Copernicus's system had a logical coherence that Ptolemy's lacked.

But there was a problem. If the massive and heavy Earth was whizzing around the Sun and spinning on its axis every day at a thousand miles an hour, surely we on Earth would be spun off into space.[11] And just think, clouds and birds would be left behind.[12] Our senses tell us we are still on Earth and, therefore, all this spinning makes no sense!

A bigger issue was that Copernicus was a canon of Frauenburg Cathedral, which meant he was one of the sixteen members of the cathedral chapter, that is, its board of directors.[13] Thus, not only did Copernicus's heliocentric cosmology defy common sense, it also ran up against the view of the Catholic Church and Psalm 104:5, "Who laid the foundations of the Earth, that it should not be removed for ever."

Copernicus proceeded cautiously, carefully concealing his data and scientific manuscript from the Church. He wrote a short report that he circulated among his closest friends. This report, called *The Commentariolus (Little Commentary),* expounded his heliocentric theory.[14] Nurturing it secretly over decades in his spare time, Copernicus advanced his blueprint for the "marvelous symmetry of the universe." In an ironic twist, one evening in 1539, a young German mathematician, Georg Joachim Rheticus, a Lutheran Protestant drawn by rumors of a celestial revolution to rival the religious upheaval of Martin Luther, stood at his door. Copernicus, now sixty-eight years old, feared his ideas would die with him.[15] Defying the Church, he let Rheticus study his discoveries. Rheticus convinced his mentor to publish his radical data.

Published in 1543, Copernicus's opus, *De revolutionibus orbium coelestium (On the Revolutions of Celestial Spheres),* was pivotal even if it was not accepted by the Church.[16] The traditional Jewish and Christian religions wrestled with traditional doctrine and the revolutionary implication about the cosmos's heliocentricity. Sooner or later, the Judeo-Christian world had to make a titanic shift in mindset and belief. No longer the center of God's Creation, the Earth became just one of the planets. By extension, this also diminished the primary position of God's highest Creation, humankind. The scale of Copernicus's heliocentric universe was earth-shaking. But crucially, it is a Truth that stands for all time. Few scientific discoveries withstand the test of time.

Copernicus was a revolutionary because he showed us that there was an intellectually respectable alternative to the accepted conception of the universe at that time. The Sun as the center of our universe is as true now as it was when Copernicus and his mentee Rheticus revealed their data.

Inevitably, someone pointed out that the evidence in Copernicus's manuscript substantiated this radical view. The Church responded: "So what?" That "someone"—Galileo Galilei—paid a heavy price:

house arrest for the last decade of his life.

Such rejection of sound science is familiar even today, is it not? We need to stop assuming that skeptical authorities necessarily have a knowledge deficit and require more facts.[17] When doubt is wrapped up in prevailing political beliefs and cultural attitudes (what Germans call the "zeitgeist"), facts often not only fail to persuade but may further entrench skepticism. Skepticism is a potent mindset that became a part of science itself. And it all started with a fiery Frenchman.

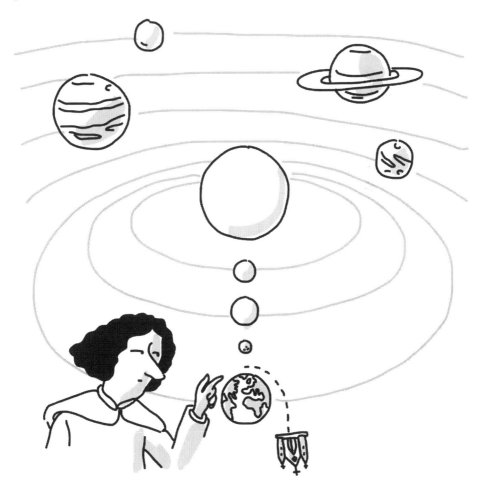

[2]
"Descartes's legacy continues to live in modern science."
A Night of Dreams and the Birth of the Miraculous Science

The date was November 10, 1619, a bitterly cold night in Ulm, Germany. A young French philosopher, his head "filled with enthusiasm," retired for the night in a stove-heated room and dreamed three dreams.[18] The first two—a pounding head and frightening visions—seemed hallucinogenic. In the third dream, René Descartes saw an encyclopedia, the famous *Corpus Poetarum Latinorum,* on a table. He opened it randomly to find counsel and stumbled on the line *Quod vitae sectabor iter?* "What path shall I follow in life?"

The next morning, Descartes duly recorded in his daily journal that his third dream revealed a vision of *"mirabilis scientiae fundamentum,"* the foundations of a marvelous science. He vowed to make a pilgrimage to the shrine of Our Lady of Loretto in thanks, for he was convinced that his dream was divine Providence. Descartes glimpsed the project that was to be his life's work. Disappointed in science, Descartes recalled "how many diverse opinions touching on the same subject matter there may be, all supported by learned men, though not more than one of them can ever be true."[19] Determined to find the truth, his self-set task from that day onward was singular: to discover a sure scientific method, based on the mathematical model, that could be applied to nature, including to animals and man.

Considering the cultural conditionings prevalent at the beginning of the seventeenth century—in particular, out-of-date ideas of science of the perceptible world, the work of Descartes appears to have been historically necessary. In addition to being a scientist and mathematician, he became a philosopher. Philosophy allowed him to reach beyond known rules. To an unprecedented degree, Descartes took the view that nature could be successfully conquered only by redescribing reality in the language of mathematics, thus purging the visual world of all that was merely visual, and then by testing these descriptions in experiments.

In *The Discourse on the Method,* one of his best-known books, Descartes boasted that his philosophy, in contrast to the Socratic tradition of questioning, critical thinking, and contemplation of Truth, is fundamentally a "practical philosophy" whose precepts yield "knowledge which is very useful in life."[20] By following his methods, Descartes wrote, we could discover the basic mechanical principles of natural phenomena and then, like skilled craftsmen, intervene and put those principles to work in the world. By so doing, he promised, in one of his most striking phrases, we could "render ourselves the masters and possessors of nature."[21]

Instead of the contemplative model of the Greeks, Descartes offered a new vision of the natural world that continues to shape our thought today: a world of matter possessing a few fundamental properties and interacting according to a few universal laws. This natural world included an immaterial mind that, in human beings, was directly related to the brain. In this way, Descartes formulated the modern version of the mind–body problem.[22] The mere fact that you think or doubt proves your own existence. His famous phrase, *Cogito ergo sum,* "I think, therefore I am," captures this ethos.[23]

As was the task of philosophy, Descartes was looking for absolute truth. To this end, he created his method of doubt. Anything that was open to doubt, he argued, could not be the absolute truth. Descartes's *Discourse on the Method* has been called the dividing line in the history of thought. Everything that came before it is old; everything that came after it is included in the formulation of the so-called "new science."[24]

What's left of Descartes today? A great deal. Descartes's influence goes far beyond algebraic notation, analytic geometry, and other mathematical innovations, such as the Cartesian coordinate system. For better and worse, the modern world is in a deep sense a Cartesian world, especially with regard to our emphasis on logic and a mechanistic interpretation of nature. To appreciate the extent of Descartes's continuing presence, consider the triumph of scientific rationality and its handmaiden, technology.[25]

If Copernicus, through his studies in astronomy, moved the stage from the center of the universe off into one of the side rooms, Descartes made us doubt *all* we see. I bestow upon Descartes a new title: *Homo dubitat,* The Man Who Doubts.

Tiller says: "Skepticism has bound up man. Beliefs shackle him down. Man is limited in his own perceptions. It started with Descartes. His method has served science for over 400 years. But man has grown, and it is time to let go of the limitations of Cartesian thought."

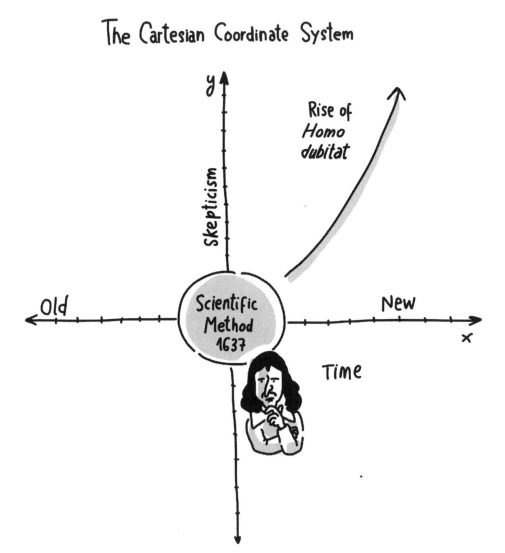

The Cartesian Coordinate System

[3]
"Medicine is stuck in chemistry."
The Pride and Prejudice of Twenty-First-Century Medicine

A letter from my present self to my younger self on graduation day from medical school, with advice that I wish I'd known about the practice of medicine:

> Congratulations, Nisha, member of the graduating class of 1991. Descartes would be proud of you! Yes, he would, for he may have been a philosopher and all that, but he said: "The preservation of health has *always* been the principal end of my studies."[26] To that end, the Cartesian agenda to promote rationalism has been magnificently carried out in medicine.
>
> When you see a patient, you see disease, something that needs to be fixed. It is a necessary part of medicine and also your patient's expectation. Yet a profound lesson you'll learn as you go along is this: Half of what you learned over the past five years (and will learn over the rest of your professional life) will be wrong. You just don't know which half.
>
> **Randomized controlled trials:** On the other hand, you are rational. Think about it: The mighty tower of modern medicine is built on rationality. And nowhere is this more evident than in the randomized controlled trial (RCT). How else can science compare what works and what doesn't? Descartes would have fully given a thumbs-up to the idea of a "dummy" or sugar pill, approving it as a "paradigm

of achieving reliable knowledge."[27] And RCT data gives reliable knowledge or evidence-based medicine, the pride of the modern medical establishment. Randomized control trials will grow in magnitude to feed medicine's excessive desire for certainty. The science of RCT and "big data" will lead to more protocols, expert guidelines, and algorithms that will preoccupy most of your clinic and free time, like an infectious case of algorithmic *education ad absurdum*.

Pharmaceuticals and new drugs: Descartes's miraculous science—to "break down each part" in hopes of becoming "masters and possessors of nature"[28] — yields new chemical medicines. Used wisely, this new knowledge will benefit your patients. But for many drug discoveries, you keep an eye out for "black box" warnings from the Food and Drug Administration (FDA). One in three drugs approved by the FDA between 2001 and 2010 were affected by significant safety issues and warnings about side effects, which were more common among drugs you prescribe.[29] You'll feel like you're standing in a banana peel universe, always about to slip on some new hazard. Never mind the problem of the dwindling number of new medications; the pharmaceutical industry has been pulling rabbits out of its hat for fifty years and is starting to run out of rabbits.[30]

Decoding the genome: In your lifetime, the whole three billion base pairs of the human genome will be decoded.[31] It's thrilling to think medicine finally has the code to life and death. Personalized medicine based on gene analysis will be hailed as the next leap to revolutionize medicine. Then you'll discover genetic analysis presents both opportunity and pitfalls. When there is only Google for your patients to check, there is room to talk them down from self-diagnosis. But when we are talking about a patient's actual genetic code, it will be difficult to convince them that "half is wrong," never mind the fact that we share a whopping 92 percent of our genetic code with mice.[32] While genes play a role in life and disease, there are innumerable epigenetic triggers that differentiate us from mice and each other. Yet genetic testing will be as cheap as buying a few coffees.

More and more pills: As Lewis Thomas, MD, pointedly wrote, over time you will watch nearly all commercials in an average evening become pitches for items to restore failed health: things for stomach gas, constipation, headaches, nervousness, sleeplessness or sleepiness, arthritis, anemia, uneasiness, the despair of malodorousness, sweat, yellowed teeth, dandruff, and piles.[33] The food industry begins to play the role of the surrogate physician, advertising breakfast cereals as though they were tonics, vitamins, and restoratives. Vitamins have taken the place of prayer. Across the pond in the UK, a person consumes, on average, a staggering forty thousand pills in a lifetime.[34]

The opioid epidemic: You will see an unprecedented opioid epidemic underway. You must use everything in your non-drug "tool bag" to help. Don't feel reluctant to openly talk about energy medicine. As he did in *Rules for the Direction of the Mind,* Descartes would wag his finger at "step by step, avoid all superfluous effort."[35] He means you must retreat and stay with what you can prove without a doubt. But you know better. Pay attention to the body's energy systems, as illustrious medical colleagues Kathi Kemper and James Oschman and qigong master healer Chunyi Lin have done.[36] Learn from them. You may not have seen energy channels in your anatomy dissection, but you're wise enough not to pooh-pooh the whole notion. The human being is complex; we just don't know everything that can be known. In fact, it's time to turn around your *Homo dubitat* self and re-examine Cartesian medicine and its answers.

The problems spelled out: You'll be seeing an excessive need for certainty with RCTs and data, and yet many medicines have problems with safety. You'll be seeing the opioid crisis. You'll see skepticism about the effectiveness of energy medicine. There is more. You'll see physician burnout, which few people talk about.[37] Many hospitals will have chief wellness officers to address fatigue and rising suicide rates among your peers.[38] Medicine will grapple with its problems incrementally, forever tinkering with incentives, education, schedules, and so on. So, what else doesn't jibe? What shall you do with a profession that will seem to have lost its way?

Stitch it back together with careful words of Truth. Chemistry alone will not restore medicine's mission of healing. You must start over, building on medical knowledge. How? With moonshot thinking. If you want to improve safety, reduce medical costs, and innovate, then don't think incrementally. Don't think 10 percent better, but ten times better. That's a mindset.[39] This isn't flash news. The highest yield for future medicine will come from fields generating the most interesting, exciting, and surprising sorts of information, most of all surprising.[40]

Using surprise as a guide, mankind progressed from Newtonian physics to electromagnetism to quantum mechanics to cosmology. And consider Barry Marshall, the hardscrabble Australian doctor who went for the moonshot, drank an infectious broth, and intentionally gave himself a stomach ulcer. He saw with fresh eyes surprising information about the presence of "corkscrew" bacteria in ulcers and solved the mystery of a deadly condition thought to be caused not by infection but by stress alone.[41]

It seems that the safest and most prudent of bets on which to lay money is surprise. There is a high probability that whatever astonishes us in biology will turn out to be usable.[42]

Take a radical new direction.

Keep faith.

Signed,

Nisha

your future self

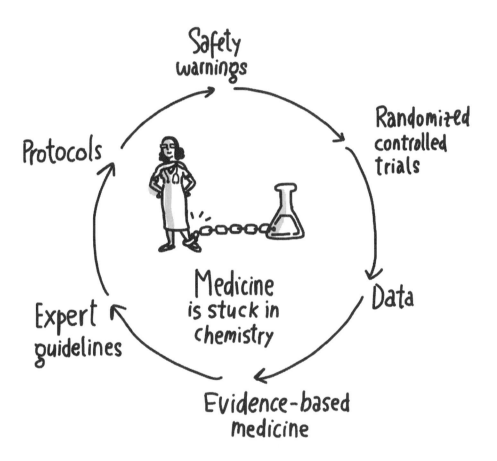

[4]
"Humans are not just chemistry.
They are a mix of energy, information,
and Spirit"
The Rise of Complementary and Integrative Medicine

Chemistry alone is insufficient for future medical progress, partly because, as Tiller puts it: "Humans are a mix. They have a physical body—the stuff of flesh and bones and matter—which medicine pays attention to, mostly. When we think in terms of a substance or physical body constructed of atoms and molecules, we also must think about an energy part, an information part, and a consciousness part. They are all part of us. The beginning is to recognize that we are all Souls and we need a body, like a suit, to experience distance–time reality. It's like a diving bell that you enter to go deep into the ocean to explore several miles down."

Tiller's description serves as a landmark in our bridge construction, and leads us to ask: How do we expand the modern medical paradigm? National statistics speak loudly: The shift in medicine is occurring as a social phenomenon. People are moving to complementary and integrative medicine (CIM), those treatments that fall outside of conventional care. Nearly one in three Americans use CIM, spending millions of dollars out-of-pocket for healthcare.[43] The main reasons they do so are disorders I see in my clinic every day: arthritis, back and neck pain, and fibromyalgia. In fact, a person with arthritis is more likely to use CIM compared to a person with heart disease or cancer.[44] It is healthcare consumers who have made a Copernican shift in collective consciousness. The basic interest in CIM in society is not led by physicians or by university professors but by patients.

With the huge numbers of adults turning to CIM, it is logical to ask what doctors feel about this. The National Institutes of Health (NIH) funded a study looking at rheumatologists' attitudes toward CIM as a treatment for the most common form of arthritis called osteoarthritis.[45] The results were surprising. Physicians had favorable views; that is, they thought therapies like massage and acupuncture and nutraceuticals like glucosamine were beneficial, and they would recommend them to their arthritic patients.

One category, however, was an outlier: energy medicine, which includes reiki, tai chi, and therapeutic touch. Compared with the other categories of CIM, rheumatologists did not believe energy medicine approaches were beneficial for osteoarthritis nor would they recommend them. Why is this? I believe major reasons are that we have no idea about the physical body's energy systems; they seem like some vague "Eastern thought." Furthermore, there is a dearth of randomized clinical trial data for reiki and tai chi in medical journals, or else it is published in little-known Chinese medical literature.

Around the same time the rheumatology survey was published, an interesting piece of original research made the front cover of the *New England Journal of Medicine* (NEJM). The NEJM is a high-impact journal considered to be highly influential in the medical field and consistently the leader in publishing cutting-edge developments in medical knowledge.[46] The randomized clinical trial investigated the effectiveness of tai chi to alleviate fibromyalgia symptoms.[47] Tai chi? In the NEJM? For something from the Eastern world to be in the NEJM was, in my mind, a game changer.

It was a game changer for several reasons. For one thing, modern medicine has few effective therapies for fibromyalgia. Here was an

RCT providing important data for energy medicine for a tough condition. This is early data, to be sure. Second, the encouraging results brought new information to doctors who may not know about tai chi and perhaps removed some of the mystery surrounding tai chi. Third, it was a catalyst for so-called nonpharmacological ways, other than prescription pain pills, to help people with chronic pain.

On this point, a search in the National Library of Medicine repository for published articles involving tai chi showed an increase from 106 articles in 2010 to 245 articles in 2018. Yet these figures are still low, underscoring that chemistry is "winning" and remains a priority in medical research. Fourth, and a related point to research, is that science could discover the mechanisms underlying tai chi. Regarding this point, I was keen to read what mechanism the authors cited for their great outcomes. After all, the NEJM would want a cause–effect theory.

As I read, I was astonished to find just one line from the study authors: "moving *qi*" was probably the reason tai chi was so effective. The article provided no explanation as to what qi is or how it "moves." Regardless, I am glad the NEJM published this work. It showed that the medical establishment can look at energy medicine, even if we don't have all the answers about what it is or why it might work.

In the second edition of the *Textbook of Complementary and Alternative Medicine,* I wrote a review of the medical literature for the effectiveness of qigong, a technique related to tai chi.[48] Reading dozens of clinical trials (including the Chinese literature when I could get it), there was a conspicuous lack of a framework for understanding energy or informational systems of the body.[49] The National Center for Complementary and Integrative Health (NCCIH) has termed the qi or energy systems of the body as the "biofield." Beyond the descriptive terms, *bio* meaning the body, and *field* implying an unseen influence extending beyond the body, there is no explanation as to what the field consists of.

Yet the qi is tangible, as my first weekend workshop at the Spring Forest qigong center in Minneapolis demonstrated to me. Unquestionably, I could feel a force of some kind, could "move" energy or qi from one part of my body to another with my intention. Master healers have pointed out that qi is the vital force of life. Whatever this biofield or lifeforce is, it exists as a component within our space–time continuum, and, as with any continuum, no endings or empty places are allowed. That is why it is called a continuum, in scientific terms, a physical field. So if lifeforce is a field phenomenon, then the science that deals with physical fields should be able to explain life, and that science is physics.[50]

Physics! Looking back, I see how I was being led to figure out the puzzle of qi from RCTs to Tillerian physics. Tiller's papers, including "Expanding the Thermodynamic Perspective for Materials in an SU(2) Electromagnetic (EM) Gauge Symmetry State Space: Part I, A Duplex Space Model with Applications to Homeopathy,"[51] talk about field aspects. When a body exerts an influence into the space around itself, physics says that the body creates a "field" around itself. Tiller uses the term "field" to convey the idea of not just the familiar electric field and gravity field, but as a description and solution to a whole new class of energies that include qi.

It was time to reset, roll up my sleeves, and bridge the gap between the all-important missing variable and unknown to medicine: the influence of fields.

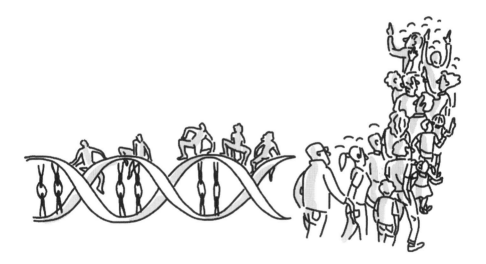

[5]
"Subtle energies are not one of the traditional forces in science."
What are Subtle Energies? The Case of Spoon Bending

The spark of electricity. It turns the compass needle. We cannot "see" the magnetic field, but we know it is present. In turn, a magnetic field induces an electric field, which induces a magnetic field, and so on. In 1864, James Clerk Maxwell, a Scottish physicist, published the nineteenth-century equivalent of a grand unified theory, which united electric and magnetic forces in the famous Maxwell's equations. Just like that, he explained light in all its varied forms: visible light, radio waves, gamma rays, and X-rays (which had not yet been discovered).

Before Maxwell, scientists had conceived of physical reality—insofar as it is supposed to represent events in nature—as material points whose changes consist exclusively of motions. After Maxwell, they conceived of physical reality as represented by continuous fields, not mechanically explicable. This change in the conception of reality was the most profound change that occurred in the study of physics.

The question is: Are qi and electromagnetism the same energy or force? Do Maxwell's equations describe qi? If qi and electromagnetism are similar forces, then standard instruments in medicine, which are designed to pick up electromagnetic signals, should be able to detect qi. But that is not what happens. Conventional tools fail to detect qi. We have the first clue: Qi does not appear to be electromagnetic.

In the 1970s, Tiller conducted experiments to test intention's capacity to direct qi.[52] With his engineering expertise, he designed a simple gas-discharge probe comprised of two thin, glass plates coated with a one-atom layer of gold metal and a two-millimeter layer of carbon dioxide and xenon mixture sandwiched between them. His device worked on the principle of gas ionization. Picture an electron in its orbit around the nucleus of a gas molecule, much like a tiny Venus around the Sun. Applying an electric current with enough energy liberates the electron, which is accelerated by the field. It collides with other gas molecules, thus freeing additional electrons. Those electrons are, in turn, accelerated.[53] The result is an avalanche multiplication. This sends off a burst of visible energy into the world, like a tiny neon light. The visible spectrum of carbon dioxide and xenon—with its lines of white, violet, blue, green, and red—can be seen in a darkened room, and the avalanche of free electrons can be heard crackling and chattering away via the speaker hooked up in series with the tube. The discharge phenomenon requires both a source of free electrons and a significant electric field to occur.

Would Tiller's subtle energy have enough power to ionize the gases? There was just one way to find out. Tiller set the gas discharge threshold such that it would be unaffected by electric forces. Thus, the system was poised but yielding a zero count until a human subject attempted to influence it. Putting his hands, palms open, about six inches from the gas discharge tube but not touching it, Tiller focused his mind on the probe, intending to increase the count rate. Over a five-minute period of such intending, the gas molecules "answered" with a series of burps, a volley of discharges of excited electrons dancing merrily, and the counter registered them going from a count of zero to the fifty thousand range. When he stood quietly by the discharge machine without intention, nothing happened. As he opened his hands and focused his mind, the burps immediately started again, unambiguously, and the device counted the discharges.

Over a two-year period, 1977 to 1979, Tiller conducted several thousand different tests with dozens of different subjects under a variety of experimental conditions. He found that almost anyone could produce a positive result—young people, old people, students, non-students, healers, nonhealers, etc., provided they had a high ability to focus their mind. If a test subject was tired or not paying attention, then the counter went quiet.

Could an alternate inanimate source also trigger the gas discharge counter? After extensive work, the answer was no. Could the human biofield be shielded from the gas discharge counter? To answer this, Tiller fitted an electrically grounded fine-mesh copper Faraday cage around the gas discharge counter. Faraday cages block electromagnetic radiation, such as radio waves and microwaves. If this idea seems strange, think of the protective grate across the window of your microwave oven. The waves that cook food in the microwave are too wide to escape through the grate, which is why the oven nukes that frozen entrée and not your hungry face. A Faraday cage works on a similar principle. Tiller found that using a Faraday cage did not lessen the discharges the counter registered. That could only mean one thing: Whatever energy was being emitted by humans to cause the enhanced counting was not a classical electromagnetic force.

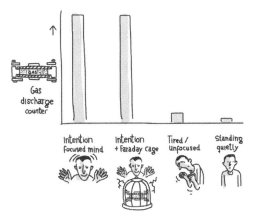

The term "subtle energy" had not yet been invented. It would enter the lexicon some years after the gas discharge work in Tiller's seminal 1993 paper "What Are Subtle Energies?"[54] At first, I found the word "subtle" misleading. Subtle, as I understand it, refers to something faint, and delicate or difficult to catch sight of and discern. My experience of subtle energy, my biofield, is anything but faint. It certainly isn't weak. This was plainly demonstrated to me.

One Thursday, Doug Matzke, a quantum physicist, joined Tiller and me in Scottsdale. Following our meeting, during lunch, Matzke was casually playing with his spoon. Suddenly, the stem of the sturdy steel metal wrapped around his finger like it was soft butter. My eyes wide, I asked: "What did you just do?"

Between chuckles, he said: "It's spoon bending. It's easy to do. You ask it 'permission' and then 'feel' the right time. Here, try it." The metal of his spoon felt like soft plastic, quickly setting into its new bent configuration. Alas, my capacity in the spoon-bending department was severely lacking. This was my first material demonstration of subtle energy doing strange things with volition.

Sometimes these spoon-bending talents seem to be completely meaningless. There is no message in a bent spoon or much practical function for it. At the same time, it invites us to consider how materials could behave like that. I made a heroic attempt to bend the framework of classical physics far enough to accommodate subtle energy phenomena. Which among the four fundamental forces could I pin my hypothesis on?

For example, we feel the consequences of gravity all the time. Matzke didn't use gravity, didn't drop his spoon from a great height onto the ground to bend the steel.

Perhaps, it is the strong nuclear force that holds protons and neutrons together. Equal, or like, charges powerfully repel each other, but the positive protons of a nucleus do not blow apart because of the "strong" force that operates at these very short distances.[55] This force obviously would not operate at the relatively gigantic distance of a steel spoon.

Then there is the phenomenon of "radioactive decay," a product of the weak nuclear force, in which atoms of certain elements "spit out" pieces of themselves and over time change into different elements. For example, uranium is radioactive and eventually turns to lead. This subatomic force is called the "weak force" and it has an even shorter range than does the "strong force."[56]

Having discounted gravity, the strong force and weak nuclear force, only one natural force recognized by science was left: electromagnetism. This is the main force acting in chemical bonds that holds bulk matter together.[57] You can hold this book or your reading device because the electromagnetic force holds the object's molecules together and your fingers don't penetrate it. So my totally materialistic interpretation of the spoon bending did not yield to what I know about electromagnetism, nor could it be classified so easily. All I could say is that some kind of human volition or intent is involved. Spoon bending's refusal to fit in with my existing knowledge was frustrating because finding patterns is how we understand nature. Famous scientists have looked at this question as well.

British physicist John Taylor, of King's College, London, became fascinated with spoon bending after witnessing it. In his book *Superminds,* he argued that a physical explanation for spoon bending could be found in electromagnetism.[58] His embrace of psychokinetic phenomena—the ability to move and change objects by mental effort alone—was replaced by skepticism when experiments conducted under laboratory conditions were negative. In Taylor's mind, an unknown fifth force with massive energy would be needed to overcome the electromagnetic forces binding the atoms together to cause steel to bend.

Taylor's dilemma was that there is no scientific evidence of such a force in physics, down through many orders of magnitude.[59] To preserve the prevailing scientific viewpoint, the idea of any fifth force had to be discarded. Taylor concluded there is no possible physical mechanism for spoon bending and other forms of psychokinesis, and it is in complete contradiction to established science.

Taylor developed a spectacular case of personal disbelief once his electromagnetic theory did not explain the phenomenon of spoon bending. I am sympathetic to Taylor, that based on his theories of electromagnetism and psychokinetics he was led to conclude that spoon bending is a hoax. I just think his was an incomplete view. I am more inclined to accept Tiller's premise that we seem to be dealing with new energy fields completely different from the ones that conventional science deals with as the basis of our present technological society. The spoon bending seems to require the presence and action of a new class of energies: "subtle" energies.

But we are just getting warmed up.

The Four Forces of Nature

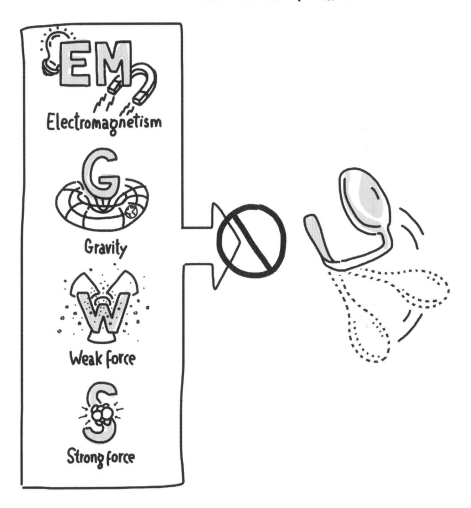

[6]
"Psychoenergetic science points the way to new possibilities for Man."
Expanding the Bounds of Subtle Energies: Psychoenergetics

Einstein reported a conversation he had with "an important theoretical physicist" regarding the relevance of research to the Einstein-Podolsky-Rosen paradox, which deals with two particles entangled with each other according to quantum mechanics.[60]

> He [physicist]: I am inclined to believe in telepathy.

> I [Einstein]: This has probably more to do with physics than with psychology.

> He: Yes.

Many scientists, including Tiller, look at psychoenergetics as real, as real as a chemical reaction in a flask, as real as the growth of salt crystals in a solution. According to Tiller, human capabilities such as telepathy, remote viewing, and clairvoyance are worthy of scientific study because they point to higher laws in the physical sciences. His aim is to give meaning to this class of human gifts. Rather than sweep these phenomena under the rug because they are difficult to prove within the accepted scientific framework, he took up the challenge and turned the principle of doubt into its opposite to show psychoenergetics prominently. I was skeptical that psychoenergetic capabilities would be of any interest to mainstream science. I couldn't have been more wrong.

Universities such as Stanford and Princeton have devoted research space and millions of dollars to investigating psychoenergetic phenomena. The science has varied in type, data collected, and degrees of effect, but they all have one thing in common: When they talk about consciousness, they talk about the ability of man to influence machines, about remote viewing, or about healing from a distance.

For example, The Princeton Engineering Anomalies Research (PEAR) laboratory under Dr. Robert Jahn and Brenda Dunne engaged in a broad range of experiments on consciousness-related anomalies. In their book *Margins of Reality: The Role of Consciousness in the Physical World,* first published in 1987, Jahn and Dunne reached provocative conclusions about the interaction of human consciousness with physical devices, such as random event generators (REG). Operators had succeeded in shifting the mean of REG in intended directions.[61]

Physicists Russell Targ and Harold Puthoff joined forces at the Stanford Research Institute (later named SRI International) in California in 1972. In their book *Mind-Reach: Scientists Look at Psychic Abilities,* they write how, in response to a request from the Central Intelligence Agency (CIA), they started and developed the remote viewing program to serve the CIA and Department of Defense (DoD) and to generate a database for scientific evaluation.[62] The research effort evolved into a highly classified, special-access program carried out under such codeword project names as "Stargate." The reports from the DoD have recently been declassified.[63]

To give you an example of the practical application of remote viewing, skilled viewer Patricia Cyrus worked closely with Stephen Schwartz and other scientists to accurately describe and locate the hiding place of Saddam Hussein in 2003.[64] Cyrus's remote viewing sketch, dated Monday, November 3, 2003, of a low building flanked on either side with trees, resembled the farmhouse under which Hussein's hiding place was located. In operation "Red Dawn" on December 13, 2003, special forces captured Hussein in Ad Dawr, fifteen kilometers southeast of Tikrit. Cyrus's remote viewing was carried out thousands of miles away in Virginia Beach, Virginia, in the United States. For this book, Cyrus provided her remote viewing results, which is included in Appendix 1.[65]

There's more. Cyrus has the ability to accurately describe and sketch news events from around the world *before* they happen.[66] Her abilities cannot be classified easily; there are no concrete features we can identify and describe scientifically to colleagues at conferences (except that now there are remote viewing conferences!). Such possibilities cannot be explained by current science, and they bring into question our understanding of spacetime. They must involve some subtle energy linkage.

It is interesting that Cyrus feels herself to be somewhat detached "between time and space" in the moments of her remote viewing and that her discipline actively encourages this condition as a method of transcending the limits of the self. Listening to her, it seems to me that we must be open to accept that individuality is not tightly circumscribed; we have to be prepared to concede that, under certain circumstances, we are "electrodes" and are potential sources and detectors of subtle energies.

What can psychoenergetics teach us about scientific revolutions? As remote viewer Lyn Buchanan writes in his book, *The Seventh Sense: The Secrets of Remote Viewing as Told by a "Psychic Spy" for the U.S. Military:* "As one person becomes more self-aware, it raises—at least a little—the level of awareness within mankind. The implications of this basic fact are enormous."[67] Maybe psychoenergetics points to a higher order in *Homo sapiens* evolution.

In the classic *Autobiography of a Yogi,* Swami Yogananda shares one of several psychoenergetic phenomena in his remarkable life: "An ecstatic enlargement of consciousness followed. I could see clearly for several miles over the Ganges River to my left, and beyond the temple into the entire Dakshineswar precincts. The walls of all buildings glimmered transparently; through them I observed people walking to and fro over distant acres."[68]

The work of Cyrus and others provide evidentiary and experiential evidence that may contribute to articulation of an epistemological underpinning for psychoenergetic phenomena. There is a reciprocal relationship between epistemology and science. They are dependent upon each other. To conclude Pillar 1, it seems appropriate to celebrate man's ingenuity and investigate a pinnacle of discovery in physics of the twenty-first century.

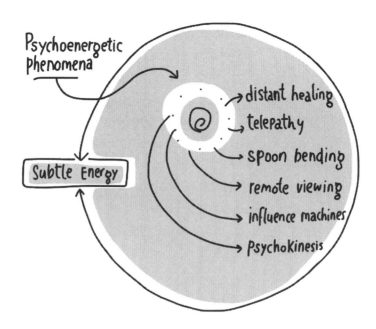

[7]
"The electromagnetic world is complete with the discovery of the Higgs boson."
God Loves Science

In the gentle, rolling hills of the French–Swiss border, more than seventeen thousand physicists ponder matter. What forces make matter behave in certain ways? Why does matter have mass? Overseeing such fundamental questions and the discovery of the whimsically named "God particle," the Higgs boson, is . . . God himself!

On June 18, 2004, the government of India gifted the *Conseil Européen pour la Recherche Nucléaire* (European Council for Nuclear Research, or CERN) in Geneva a six-foot bronze statue of Shiva Nataraja, "dancing Shiva," symbolizing the cosmic dance of creation and destruction.[69] Lord Shiva is encircled by a ring of flames that are "not of fuel." It is a metaphor beyond perfect, for buried three hundred feet into the ground below the statue is a ring of "fire," also not of fuel, created by man with more than forty thousand tons of superconducting magnets. This ring, the Large Hadron Collider or LHC, is the most powerful and colossal particle accelerator on Earth.[70]

The energies and force field of the LHC magnets recreate the "fire" of the primordial Big Bang. Two beams of protons in opposite streams whirl around the twenty-seven-kilometer ring, propelled by the tremendous magnetic force. The circular design creates an infinitely long distance through which the proton beam may be accelerated; particles travel through the same system continuously, accelerating faster and closer to the speed of light.

Above ground, Shiva holds a rattle drum, the *damaru,* constructed of two cones meeting at their points. Imagine: as Shiva's damaru resounds, the LHC magnets start up. Shiva dances, his left foot and left hand elegantly raised to signify movement in the cosmos. Underground, a six-teraelectronvolt magnetic field energizes the protons with herculean power. Shiva's damaru reverberates louder. The speed of the particles is intensified by the LHC's accelerating structures. Protons dance in the beams, as though urged by God, thundering, powerful, and intense, at 99.99 percent the speed of light. Shiva's hair whirls with the energy and ecstasy of his dance. Quadrupole magnets focus protons into a concentrated beam, the width of a hair, which whirl around the ring of fire at eleven thousand revolutions per second.

Suddenly, the beams meet head on, like the cone points. Shiva's right foot crushes the dwarf of ignorance. Protons slam together at energies of 13 trillion electron volts and, amid the roar and lightning, are annihilated. For a flicker—just 10^{-22} seconds—a new form of matter is created, disappearing into mists in the chambers of super-cooled helium. The Higgs boson has been found, as was predicted by the standard model of matter.

What does the confirmation of the Higgs boson really signify?

Tiller explains: "The discovery of the Higgs boson is an important discovery. It signals the closure of the electromagnetic world. All the boxes in the standard model have been filled. Nature is much richer than electromagnetism (EM). It is time to march ahead beyond the EM science."

The standard model description of nature is incomplete in important ways. It turns out that what we call "normal matter," which is things like protons and the Higgs boson, barely makes up *5 percent* of the Universe. What is the other 95 percent made of? We don't know.[71]

We turn to Shiva for answers.

"O Omnipresent, the embodiment of all virtues, the creator of this cosmic universe, the king of dancers, who dances the Ananda Tandava in the twilight, I salute thee," chants a verse from the Sivanandala-hari, inscribed on the CERN plaque.[72]

A knowing smile plays on Shiva's tranquil face. He reveals that ultimate reality has no form, no matter. Accordingly, Shiva is showing us that transcendent Truth is beyond the speed of light! This limit—a sacred cow of physics—is not fundamental, intrinsic, integral, or indivisible reality. By extension, humans are part of nature and any description of nature includes us. Humankind's roots belong in the superluminal realms.

Tiller says: "All of the important stuff of us, the soul-self stuff where we truly are one, is in the superluminal domain and therefore looks invisible to us and to our instruments because they are made from electromagnetic waves, which are subluminal. You cannot perceive them with [those kinds of] instruments. That's the old world for us."

Can science dispense altogether with the idea of matter? It seems likely to prove a more fruitful starting point for investigation of consciousness. Can science take us beyond the speed of light?

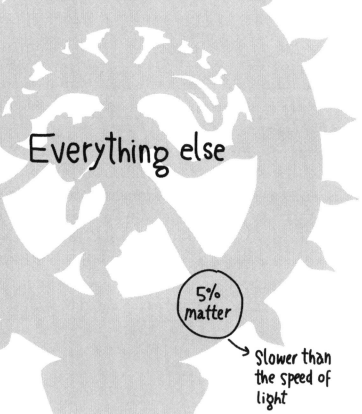

What price do you offer for an antique bridge whose principal assets are legend, architectural beauty, quality granite, and a song handed down from generation to generation reporting the bridge's antecedent is falling down?

—Roger A. Johnson

New City, Old Bridge Bridge, made in reference to London Bridge [73]

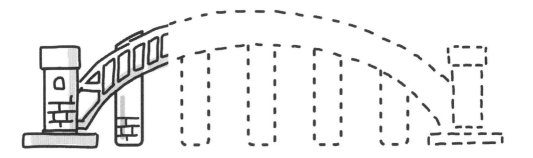

BRIDGE PILLAR 2:
Mind Beyond Brain and Levels of Being

Our physical science does not necessarily deal with reality, whatever that is. Rather, it has merely generated a set of consistency relationships to explain our common ground of experience, which is determined, of course, by the capacity and capabilities of our physical sensory-perception mechanisms.

–WILLIAM A. TILLER[74]

[8]
"Consciousness is not localized in your brain."
The Tyranny of Brain Science

We are witnessing a great era of consciousness research in academia. In 2013, the US federal government teamed up with the European Union and announced ambitious endeavors to promote and integrate future brain research.[75] The National Institutes of Health (NIH) laid out a blueprint for neuroscience to boost neurobiology research and technology through a series of focused objectives and "grand challenges" to scientific investigators.[76] During the period from 2010 to 2018, entries associated with keywords "brain" or "neuron" in the US National Library of Medicine, the definitive index of life science publications, grew steadily from thirteen thousand per year in 1970 to more than sixty thousand per year. Bibliometric studies of the "hot spots" in neuroscience publications between 2006 and 2015 show that the terms "autism" and "neuro-imaging" were among the most frequently cited.[77] Attendance at the annual American Academy of Neurology conference in 2018 topped fourteen thousand, surpassing the population of some entire towns in America.

With such concentration of monies and intellectual brain power devoted to three kilograms of gray tissue housed in the human skull, one of the greatest problems that must be overcome in the development of a scientific theory of consciousness is the idea of the brain as the source of consciousness. The problem, as I see it, is that there seems to be something special about functional magnetic resonance imaging (fMRI) that elevates brain images to the status of a law. Neuroscientific theories about the working of the brain assume that for one to "feel" or "decide," it is necessary that one activates their brain. Discussions of consciousness are framed solely in terms of brain signals, trillions of synapses creating us as an emotional and feeling species, that is, with phenomenal consciousness. The principle of neuroplasticity is embedded in the data and gives rise to the popular slogan "Happiness is learned."

Yet some researchers caution us about brain imaging. In his book *The Biological Mind: How Brain, Body, and Environment Collaborate to Make Us Who We Are,* neuroscientist Alan Jasanoff warns us that brain-scanning technologies are still in their infancy and provide only crude and ambiguous data; yet the beautiful, colorized pictures from such scans are taken as a microcosmological map of our inner lives.[78] Slowly but surely, brain science has become holy writ.

We must talk about what the textbooks don't say. They don't say anything about what the brain MRI *means.* To get at what cognitive scientist David Chalmers calls the "hard problem" of consciousness,[79] the difficulties have nothing to do with brain anatomy and physiology. The difficulties of mind are conceptual. Consider that brain anatomy and physiology do not give rise to my elation of seeing my favorite shade of blue or tasting Kenyan coffee. It is interesting to know that someone produces a special set of brain-wave functions while bending a stainless-steel spoon, but I don't believe it means any more than the observation that his hands perspire while he is thinking about that special someone. The measurements are purely symptomatic and tell us nothing about the spoon, the special someone, or one's own relationship to his consciousness. Looking for physical explanations of consciousness is like attacking a piano with a sledgehammer to get at the concerto imprisoned inside.[80] It's a maniacal endeavor.

Relying on anatomy, we are reduced to the view that "I-ness" and the "self" are both illusions, particular sensations created by material consequences of material neurons and their material chemical and electrical activities. We are nothing but a bunch of atoms and molecules. Where does that leave us?

Also, we don't know how far down anatomy of the brain one must go to the source of consciousness. Down to the level of cells? To the levels of the cell membrane? Or maybe the DNA? Yet, as you unravel the proteins of the double helix, all they do is spin and vibrate. Your DNA cannot write Beethoven's *Fifth Symphony*.

Perhaps we will have to look to the molecular level. For example, it was only recently discovered that a quantum process is necessary for photosynthesis. I expect that we will find the same is true for some aspects of what goes on between our ears. Currently, theories posit that quantum events in the brain create consciousness.[81] But no one has credibly shown how molecules learned to think, that is, to perform cognition accompanied by conscious experience.

We must not forget the neurons in our guts, including how the brain, the gut, and the trillions of microorganisms living in our gut communicate with each other. Your gut is like a supercomputer. While medicine has long viewed the digestive system as largely independent of the brain, we now know that these two organs are intricately connected with each other, as reflected in the concept of the gut–brain axis. Based on this concept, our digestive system is much more delicate, complex, and powerful than we once assumed. Recent studies suggest that, in close interactions with its resident microbes, the gut can influence our basic emotions, our pain sensitivity, and our social interactions. It even guides many of our decisions![82]

This is all very well, but we are still missing the point. Consciousness is not temporal or spatial. It isn't housed in a skull or the gut or even the gut's Lilliputian army. The brain is an impressive, adaptive wiring system, as wiring systems go. Brain scientists have many arguments to deflect the charge of the limitations of anatomy and imaging as the basis for modeling human consciousness. I am reminded of how language also shapes our perceptions of nature. "If I ask about the world," wrote Nelson Goodman, a Harvard philosopher, "you can offer to tell me how it is under one or more frames of reference; but if I insist that you tell me how it is apart from all frames, what can you say? We are confined to ways of describing whatever is described. Our [perception of the] universe, so to speak, consists of these ways rather than of a world."

Tiller said: "Experts have a 'boggle-eye effect' when considering a model of consciousness without a brain."

Books by people who have had near-death experiences—such as one by neurosurgeon Eben Alexander, talk about one thing: Consciousness is not in the brain.[83] Being both nontemporal and nonspatial, consciousness isn't "housed" in your head. Are your synapses starting to misfire? The following story illustrates how science is using a "better light over here" in the skull.

The Sufi master Mullah Nasruddin was on his hands and knees searching for something under a streetlamp.[84] A man saw Nasruddin and asked, "What are you looking for?"

"My house key. I lost it."

The man joined him in searching for the key, and after some time of fruitless searching, the man asked, "Are you sure you lost it around here?"

"Oh, I didn't lose it around here. I lost it over there, by my house."

"Then why are you looking for it over here?"

"Because," Nasruddin said, "the light is much better over here." We need a new brainstorm. Or a better light.

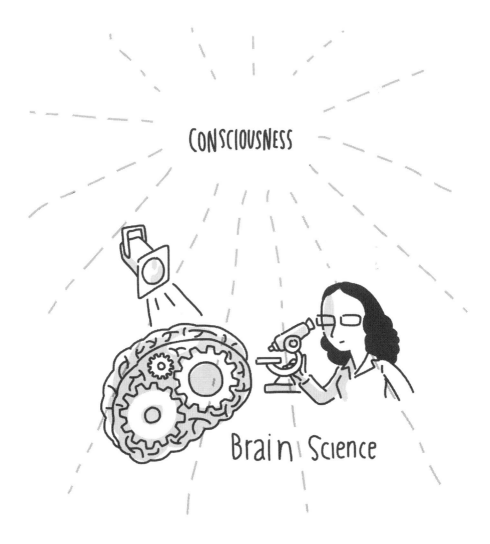

[9]
"To thine own self be true."
Can a Robot Have Consciousness?

Regarded by many as possibly the wisest man who ever lived, I see Socrates as a role model for the exploration of consciousness because he spoke freely about his experiences. The Socratic method laid the groundwork for Western systems of logic and philosophy. This method is a different style of education than a lecture and involves a conversation between a teacher and a student who is asked to question his or her assumptions. For example, we could have a debate back and forth about the relationship between consciousness and the body. Even if we don't know the answers, it does lead into another interesting question: How do people think the two are connected? This is where "experimental philosophy" comes in.[85]

Instead of the traditional method of philosophical debates, the new field of experimental philosophy uses methods of contemporary cognitive science: questionnaires, statistical analyses, data modeling, and so on. In other words, in modern-day philosophy, the scientist is leaving the armchair, so to speak.

A number of scientists have been employing experimental philosophy to plumb people's intuitions about consciousness. Suppose you look around and notice two objects, the TV remote and your goldfish in a bowl.[86] How do you decide which of these two items has consciousness? Like most people, you have a clear intuition about the answer: the goldfish. Experimental philosophy says when people are trying to determine whether an entity is capable of having mental states, its behavior guides us. The goldfish demonstrates complex behaviors such as swimming around and chomping on fish food and has a living, breathing body. The TV remote, on the other hand, does not have apparent conscious behaviors.

In the second experiment, you are given a robot and a human. The robot is constructed of metal, silicone, and rubber; it looks and behaves like a human in every way. Does the robot have two eyes and a mouth? Yes, you answer. Then it gets more interesting. How about: "Is the robot happy when it gets what it wants?" Your response to this question is a resounding no. The robot may function and look physically like a human—it walks on two legs, has the right kind of face, and even talks to you about the weather, but you refuse to believe that it can possess phenomenal consciousness like being happy, sad, or joyous. Why is that?

What we really want to know is why people have the intuitions they do, giving us a view into internal psychological processes.[87] This leads to a surprising aspect of people's intuitions about whether a robot is actually capable of feeling anything. If people are asked about a robot that has a computer processing unit (CPU) in his head but an ordinary human body, then they are significantly more likely to say that this robot could have feelings. In other words, it seems like people think the ability to have feelings depends in some fundamental way on having the *right kind of a body*.[88] Specifically, it appears that ascribing states of phenomenal consciousness shows a special sort of sensitivity to purely *physical factors*. Experimental philosophy studies point to the fact that our biases about what can and cannot possess consciousness seem to be tied to the right kind of face and flesh and bones and brain.

Returning to objects like a TV remote having consciousness, we ask: "Is it a closed question?" As noted by Isaac Newton's biographer

Richard Westfall: "The ultimate cause of atheism is this notion of bodies having, as it were, a complete, absolute and independent reality in themselves."[89]

There may be a way out of this; it may turn out that consciousness is a much more generalized mechanism, shared not only among ourselves but with all the other conjoined things of our Universe. Since perhaps we are not so absolutely central, we may be able to get a look at it, but we will need new technology for this kind of neurobiology. In that case, we will likely find that we have a whole eternity of astonishment stretching out ahead of us.

In the meantime, we would be wise to follow the Socratic injunction of *know thyself.*

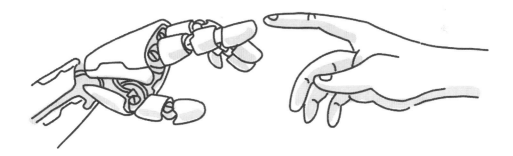

[10]
"Your unconscious mind is a powerhouse."
Your Conscious Mind Is Mostly Asleep

With the many tasks I must attend to on a daily basis, I can barely attend to more than one object at a time, and I can hardly perform two tasks at once. So to somehow enhance my cognitive capabilities, I try meditation and sleep, along with a cup or two of good coffee. Walking down my local supermarket aisle to the coffee section, I noted how we all covet better brains. I passed the section stocking brain nutrition and vitamins. Bars to improve your focus. Bars to keep you awake. From the perspective of better concentration, there were brain-training puzzles at checkout. It seems everyone wants a piece of the action. Attention as an aspect of consciousness is enshrined elsewhere and everywhere as an element of reliability.

Pause for a moment and consider: Do you notice the pressure of the chair on your back, or the speck of dust that just floated merrily in front of your face, or that bird song outside your window? Literally billions of pieces of information are flooding your senses every millisecond, but you don't consciously perceive it all. That is probably a good thing, to avoid overwhelming your attention. Speaking of attention, what is going on in your mind right this moment? Most of what goes on in your mind is not conscious. Little of human life can be genuinely described as conscious.

Open any medicine textbook and turn to the neurology chapter. Almost without exception, there is the glaring omission of a startling fact: Your brain processes a minuscule amount of information.[90] These textbooks repeat a conclusion reached in the 1950s that has been repeated sporadically in the medical and psychological literature, yet without making much of an impact either on physiology and neuropsychology or on our culture as a whole.[91] The brain receives about eleven million pieces (known as bits in information theory) of information per second from sensory sources, but conscious thought can handle, at most, forty bits per second. An awful lot is going on that you do not notice.

In his book tellingly titled *The User Illusion: Cutting Consciousness Down to Size,* science writer Tor Nørretranders writes that our brain presents us with a user interface much like a computer does: delayed in time, compressed, summarized, edited, and incomplete.[92] Every one of us discards millions of bits of information to arrive at what we term "conscious perception." Our survival depends on unconscious decisions; in fact, conscious perception lags at least half a second behind events. Nørretranders writes that your brain makes decisions at least a half second before "you" think "you" have made a decision. We exist in a user illusion.

Many of our behaviors, phobias, neuroses, psychoses, and human interactions can be analyzed in terms of this powerful illusion. The subconscious, on the other hand, can process millions of bits of information per second. The thesis is straightforward, at least when expressed in numbers. There are many skills that we carry out without thinking about what we are doing. Someone can play the piano without being aware of every aspect of it. The vast majority of processing is accomplished outside conscious notice and most of the body's activities take place outside direct conscious control. Even as "simple" an activity as walking is best done without interference from consciousness, which does not have enough information-processing capability to keep up with the demands of this task.[93]

Tiller says of consciousness: "The unconscious is gathering all the information and processing it and in doing so generates small kernels of information, which it sends to your conscious mind so that the conscious mind will know it is alive. Furthermore, your unconscious only sends them along pathways the conscious mind has given meaning. If the conscious mind does not give meaning to the information, it is basically 'dumped.' If you want to grow, give things meaning. Expand your conscious bandwidth."

In his book *Blink,* social science writer Malcolm Gladwell says our unconscious is a powerful force processed by the brain.[94] For example, an art expert can make a decision about the authenticity of a painting by relying on the unconscious processing of vast amounts of information in a few seconds and arrive at the correct answer without consciously gathering facts and evidence about the art at hand. Learning to understand and program our unconscious is one of life's important and integral purposes.

Readers might have noted that I along with Mr. Gladwell have fallen into the same trap of thinking that these super-fast perceptions happen due to brain "processing." Mea culpa. The unconscious mind is powerful, but I don't believe it is because of the wiring in our brain; rather it is the concept of "everywhereness" that psychoenergetic science has pointed out.

Something like a field effect is at play.

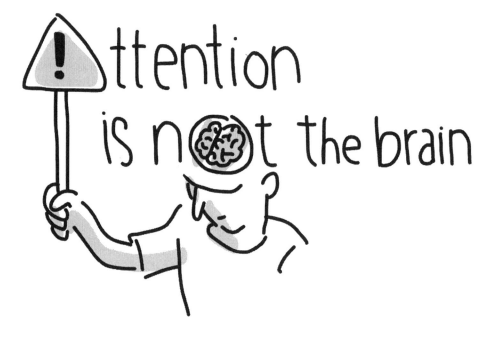

[11]
"Consciousness is a continuum of levels."
Levels of Being and the Map of Consciousness

We will assign a valid meaning to the idea of consciousness. Logically, no two things, creatures, and persons are the same. The notions of differences in consciousness involve some sort of measurement.

In his seminal book *A Guide for the Perplexed*,[95] British economist Ernst Friedrich Schumacher offered a scale he called "Levels of Being," consisting of four great levels: the mineral world, the plant world, the animal world, and finally humans. Each level contains the essence of the levels below it. For example, plants have minerals, *m*, but also a factor *x*, because a plant grows and has life. An animal has mineral *m*, as well as life *x*, but has a jump in powers compared with a plant because of the quality Schumacher labels as *y*, signifying consciousness. Animals like dogs and cats have the quality of consciousness. Man has a jump in powers, for he has a capability that surpasses even the most highly developed animals. Man has the powers of life like a plant, powers of consciousness like the animal, and something more: an ability to think. Schumacher labeled the quality of "thinkingness" as *z*.

$$Man = m + x + y + z$$
$$Animal = m + x + y$$
$$Plant = m + x$$
$$Mineral = m$$

Schumacher's characterization of "lower" and "higher" Levels of Being opens the door to ideas of evolution or development, as well as freedom. Consciousness imparts evolution as expressed in thinking-ness. This quality of thinkingness, z, that man possesses must also be expanded to show the range of his thoughts, from what we universal-ly accept as negative, such as deception or jealousy, to positive ones, such as willingness and love. As literary theorist Geoffrey Hartman wrote, "There are as many consciousnesses or *cogitos* as there are individuals."[96]

There are no instrument measurements available to us. How-ever, medical scientist and mystic Dr. David Hawkins arrived at a semi-quantitative measurement of man's thoughts with muscle test-ing, also known as kinesiology. Hawkins's choice of kinesiology was inspired by holistic physician John Diamond's work detailed in his classic book, *Your Body Doesn't Lie: How to Increase Your Life Ener-gy through Behavioral Kinesiology*.[97] Kinesiology is like dowsing or divining, discovering the unknown and hidden condition of physical health through the muscle response and without utilizing scientific apparatus.

Conventional medicine does not make use of kinesiology. On the other hand, many integrative healers use kinesiologic muscle testing in diagnosing physical ailments. My observations of the clinical prac-tices and methods of kinesiology by chiropractor, Dr. Edward Wagner and licensed acupuncturist Steven Tonsager illustrates that they use both inspiration and knowledge in their practices.[98] Using kinesiolo-gy in their clinics, they, it seems to me, arrive at a point where phys-ical and spiritual forces combine to produce the answer; in this case, truth about the health of a patient. Their full clinics attest to the pow-er of their methods, reaching into regions where conventional care cannot hope to go, such as patients' unconscious patterns.

A diviner has to discriminate between "yes" (e.g., muscle contracts and stays strong) and "no" (e.g., muscle relaxes and weakens) responses to information.[99] This is a subtle energy effect. No known physical process can explain why dowsing aids such as pendulums, amber beads, or brass rods are effective as amplifiers. Indeed, the variety of aids suggests that they are in themselves unimportant. The vital component in dowsing and muscle tests is a *human being*. An indispensable guide to the subject is Hawkins's book *Power versus Force. The Hidden Determinants of Human Behavior.*[100]

Hawkins's Map of Consciousness® is a continuous numerical scale from zero, for nonliving or dead, to a thousand, signifying the highest levels of consciousness, such as that of masters like Christ and Buddha. It is a logarithmic scale, which means that each one-point ascent on the scale is an increase in power by a factor of 10. The advantage of the map is that it gives us the ability to place consciousness in the context of the hierarchic structure of the world; it gives us a way to distinguish between higher and lower consciousness.

On the map, medicine occupies the world of the intellect. Medicine is about mechanisms, deductions, and diagnoses. Intellect serves it well; with intellect, medicine has formed theories and laws around the physical body. The map allowed me to see the dynamics of medicine and its relationship to other levels. For example, medicine can be uncomfortable with ideas of love or spirituality, which are significantly higher on the scale. The intellectual level is more familiar and comfortable for physicians.

An important aspect of Hawkins map is the idea of discernment. Many times, my conscious perception is not able to sort out truth from rubbish. The map can serve as a method to distinguish between the two using muscle testing as an indicator of truth versus falsehood. It might be useful in reading this book, for example, to validate whether what I write about is truthful or rubbish.

For now, I'll give an example. While researching qi and learning more about Tiller's work on intention, I came to feel strongly an urge to investigate the feeling of wonder reading his indecipherable paper. His book *Psychoenergetic Science,* including its cover, title, and content, all read like a lab manual. I had to be sure that his science is truthful. How could I do that? During the question and answer session of David Hawkins seminar in Prescott, Arizona, I asked Hawkins about Tillerian physics and its level on the Map of Consciousness. To 'get at' whether *Psychoenergetic Science* was valid and in integrity, Hawkins muscle tested his partner Susan Hawkins with verbal information about the level of truth of Tiller's book. Astonishingly, this book has a level of consciousness at 575—and Susan's muscle stays strong.

That number—575—surpasses the intellect and is well into the realm of the heart. There was a whole level of science, not what I had learned from textbooks and lectures in medical school and not even what I had learned as a medical doctor, but a level I had hardly ever conceived. Science and Love? Yes, they can work together.

Another lesson for me: Don't judge a book by its cover.

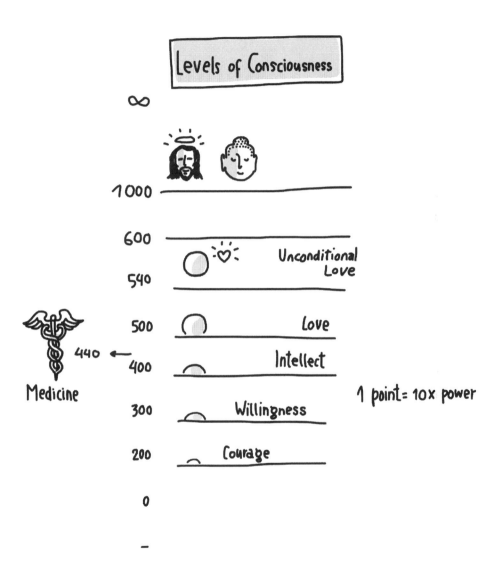

[12]
"Intention is a process of creation.
But first, you have to clear out your crap."
By Intention, Your Consciousness Creates

Tiller investigates what consciousness is by asking about consciousness operationally, about what consciousness does. He gives it a practical question. Your consciousness *does* things by intention.

Tiller understands that having a clear, focused intention requires a steady mind, honed by meditation. Meditation helps to reduce internal noise by clearing out the crap, those incessant mental objects of thinkingness. I must admit, when he used the word "crap" it was meant as a kindly jolt to me. To wake me up, like a Zen master's treatment of young disciples to encourage clearer understanding of their wandering minds.

Tiller's word "crap" also brought to my mind the classic allegory of a famed Zen teaching: Searching for the Ox. Having become oriented to the nature of the work before me in order to clear my cluttered and noisy mind, I must begin to truly do it. The work can be painful and slow, like taming an ox. Once I see my patterns and habits, these can be unlearned so that I can realize wisdom in my intention and actions.[101]

Intention pervades our life: every day, every moment, entirely. It determines how you dress, what you eat for breakfast, which car you drive, the movies you enjoy, and how you marshal your thoughts, which ones fly away, and which grab your conscious attention. Intention, like oxygen, is something we take for granted; it is unseen, can seldom be fully imagined, and is rarely properly discussed. Your intention is a product of a variety of personal, cultural, and even philosophical forces all woven together.

One more thing must be added to this definition: the concept of creation. The moment of creative discovery is a crucial one. From a deeper, more profound level, thought is stimulated, or perhaps more correctly, fed to the conscious mind, and intention is strengthened. Creation is especially important because of the operational process of intention. An operation is about taking action and therefore forms an active principle of this book. Through creation, intention is rendered testable, a felt thing, even though it is intangible and cannot be seen.

Intention is all around us. Think of all the ordinary objects around you. Have you ever taken a good look at a public garbage can in London, a paving stone in Mexico City, or a doorway in Mumbai? The man or woman responsible for making those utilitarian objects started with intent, then got busy creating.[102] Intention, dedication, and perseverance come together, and the results can be something astonishing. Sometimes the work even achieves immortality.

As I went about my morning, I brushed my teeth with a toothbrush, used a safety pin to find a drawstring, put on my sandals, and tucked my bamboo fork in my bag. Then I thought about sliced bread, cheese, tomato, and mayo. Suddenly there is a masterpiece cheese and tomato sandwich, a creation that endures in memory. Intention is behind it all, hidden but at work right now in your heart and mind, asking for recognition, asking to be given meaning.

That the principle of creation is interwoven with intention prompts a general philosophical question: What is the motivation behind intention? Perhaps not literally or perfectly, but it is like having a feeling and then putting it into words in a poem. The words might not fully encompass the emotion, but the words are a great representation of what was intended.

It also helps you learn from the observation of your subconscious subjective activities, which are concerned with the actual evolution of your instrument of consciousness. To achieve this, you must first give your attention to your subconscious activities. You must amplify them. Concentrate on them. Attention of the senses, mind, and soul, amplification of individual processes—the contemplative, analytical, and creative are all brought into play.

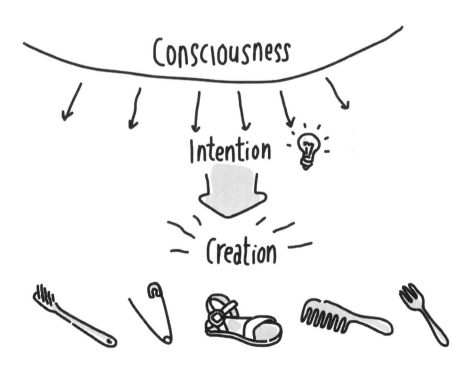

[13]
"We have to go beyond space-time when we consider consciousness."
Science Beyond Spacetime

Sometimes the hard part is identifying our assumptions, especially when they seem natural and straightforward. So it is with space and time. "Beyond spacetime" may sound like a ridiculous idea, but it has good precedent in spiritual texts.[103]

Time. I am ruled by it: schedules, meetings, appointments, running out of time with the manuscript of this book. Books have been devoted to the question of whether time is real or an illusion. I settled on the all-time bestseller *A Brief History of Time* by Stephen Hawking.[104] Alas, my time was not well spent on this read. Of the 200 pages, just two pages are relevant to the history of time. Thus, only one percent of the book can be said to be faithful to its title. Hawking's book is really *A Brief History of Science.*

I wondered what another ultra-famous cosmologist had to say about time. In formulating his theory of special relativity, Einstein tackled the concept of time. He realized that to address the paradox that the speed of light is a universal constant, appearing the same to moving observers, he would need to re-pose the philosophical question "What is time?" in an operational form: "What must you do to *measure* time?" In analyzing this question, Einstein showed that different observers, moving with respect to one another, arrive at different definitions of time. For example, to a stationary observer, a clock that is moving relative to him will be measured to tick slower than a clock that is at rest in his frame of reference. This case is sometimes referred to as special relativistic time dilation.

Cosmology and the concept of time got me thinking. What does it mean to ordinary folks like you and me? I frequently fly across time zones, and my BlackBerry adjusts to the new local time automatically. It seems to "know" Earth's revolutions, day and night. Time flew by just thinking about time. Time is money and we are wasting time. Are you having the time of your life reading this or is time standing still? The concept of time is truly cultural. I am Indian, and Indians sometimes tease each other about having "Indian Standard Time": Nothing is set in concrete clock-time. So people arrive "late" for occasions, but they are actually on time, according to Indian Standard Time, that is.

When we talk about time flow, about whether time is running fast or slow, we do not mean time *itself* is running. Events *change* and unfold in time. It turns out that our clock is between our ears. Science suggests that the best language for thinking about nature is that of change, not of permanence. How does one describe nature in which everything occurs but there is no time variable? Actually, to describe nature, as theoretical physicist Carlo Rovelli writes in his book *The Order of Time,* a time variable is not required. What is required are variables that *describe* time: quantities that we can perceive, observe, and measure. The length of a road, the height of a plant, the temperature of a forehead.[105]

Profoundly, Rovelli also asserts (and I agree) that time is about *becoming*. It speaks to evolution, to higher states of consciousness, which, in this space we call home, takes time. We evolve as we think and intend and create. We evolve in how we interact in our relationships with each other. We understand the world and our place in it by *becoming*.[106]

The time has come to start over in how we think about space. Einstein showed that space is not abstract. Instead, think of it like a dynamic, flexible rubber sheet. It is a physical thing that can bend (in the presence of massive objects), ripple (called gravitational waves), or expand.[107] I doubt these cosmological fascinations occupy the minds of even a tiny fraction of people. But it is worthwhile to pause now and consider space.

We cannot see it, touch it, or feel it with any of our senses, as most people will say. I challenge this type of limited thinking. Most people imagine space as emptiness in which events happen. In this view, space is literally the absence of things. It is a void waiting to be filled, as in "I saved space for dessert" or "I found a great parking space." Beyond everyday usage to convey emptiness, notice we often use spatial qualities to illustrate something deeper: Spatial dimensions are invoked to describe admirable qualities. Consider this: I may say that Tiller has reached *great heights* or has immense *depth*. What about doing *inner* work or a heart *expanding* with joy? All of these are attributes to do with space.

Space is not a static empty backdrop on which the theater of our lives plays out. American physicist, mathematician, and philosopher Franklin Merrell-Wolff writes in his exemplary book *Pathways Through to Space* that "Space is Divine."[108] You are familiar with the three-dimensional spaces in your home—kitchen, living room, bedrooms—and they all have their distinct *ambience* or *quality*. What else can space do? Perhaps, like water, space has different states and properties and phases. Maybe it can rearrange itself in weird ways or have totally unexpected properties, the same way that water behaves differently when it is a liquid, a solid, or a vapor. Maybe there are other types of space in our universe.

So space and time are in no way absolute. Space and time are a convenient way to write laws in a form suitable for calculations. The relation of mathematics and equations to reality suggests that these somehow belong to the fabric of the universe rather than being generated by human attempts to understand it. But deeper properties of consciousness, as psychoenergetics has shown, appear to be beyond space and time. New means of measurement are needed to fill the gaps in systems of equations. For now, for calculations, the concepts of space and time are useful.

Space can do surprising things:

Space

Expand

Bend

Ripple

and more to be discovered…

[14]
"There must be a mathematical formalism between intention and experiment that can be directly tested and quantified."
Inner Workings of a Physicist: *Adaequatio*

In the movie *Hidden Figures,* set in the early 1960s, the then-director of NASA Al Harrison remarks to Katherine Johnson, a "computer" running the numbers of the orbits of the Earth and moon: "I want all my geniuses to look beyond the numbers, to look around them, through them, for answers to questions we don't even know to ask. Math that doesn't yet exist. Because without it, we're not going anywhere. We are staying on the ground. We're not flying into space, we're not circling the earth, and we're certainly not touching the moon. And in my mind, in my mind, I'm already there. Are you?"[109]

In 2019, we are struggling with the science of consciousness. Can we look beyond the brain images, look through the colorful pictures, look around them for answers to questions we don't even know to ask? To search for a testable theory that doesn't yet exist? Because without it, we are stuck in our skulls. We are not going anywhere, and science is not contributing to human evolution, other than technological prowess and daily comfort. It is not contributing to our level of *becoming.*

I know what you're thinking. Hasn't quantum mechanics provided an answer to consciousness? Science is about tools. In physics, equations are tools that describe and predict behaviors and phenomena in nature. There are many kinds of equations in quantum mechanics, but one type is especially important: differential equations.

Such equations involve concepts from calculus, and instead of dealing directly with some physical quantity they describe how quantities change with time.[110] More precisely, they specify the *rate of change* of a physical quantity. For example, take a hot cup of coffee. As it cools down, the rate of heat lost to the air is different at each point in time as it cools. At first, the rate of change of coffee temperature will be steep. As it cools, the temperatures of the coffee and room become closer, and the rate of change of coffee cooling should decrease. The rate of cooling of coffee is a function of the relationship of its temperature, the room temperature, and time.

In quantum mechanics, the Schrödinger equation is especially important. As a partial differential equation, the Schrödinger equation is used to find the allowed energy levels of atoms. The associated wavefunction gives the probability of finding a particle at a certain physical position with time. To show consciousness effects on subatomic particles, we must have an equation to solve. But there is no differential equation for consciousness. There appears no way to directly test any hypothesis of intention with quantum mechanics and arrive at a mathematical formula.

Then why bother with physics? We have no tools, no mathematical equations with which to study consciousness, and besides, the airy-fairy notion of "beyond spacetime" leaves us at an impasse. The assertion that intention effects can never be predicted from first principles is a self-fulfilling prophecy, because it discourages us from the hard work necessary to pursue the problem to its limit.

This brings us to an idea posited by Schumacher in *A Guide for the Perplexed:* What gives even *physical* sciences the ability to make predictions? What enables man to know anything at all about the world around him? "Knowing demands the organ fitted to the object," said Greek philosopher Plotinus. Nothing can be known without an appropriate instrument in the constitution of the knower. This is the great truth which defines knowledge as *adaequatio rei et intellectus:* The understanding of the knower must be adequate to the things to be known. Science rarely discusses the qualifications or *adaequatio* of the scientist.[111]

Tiller vaults over the mathematics in the interest of practicality. Practical intentions matter as much as, if not more than, purely mathematical ones. This is an engineer's mindset; math is a means to an end. He knows mathematics and, importantly, is able to invent whatever he needs. He builds connections of detached branches of science through overarching principles using word equations.

We may protest and say that words are imprecise and too limited, too colored by assumptions to provide a route to deeper aspects of reality. Yet, I would argue, it is his leaning toward using language that gives Tiller strength and an edge. Word equations form a bridge from the subtle world to the material world, and later the data is generated by experiments. Words and verbal communication in science can be traced from the days of the Greek tradition of Pythagoras and Archimedes. Word equations have power. Power is in the equal sign. Equations are a way to working out the value and equivalence of some quantity. An equation is a kind of puzzle centered on a hypothesis.

Tiller's hypothesis centered on intention and on subtle energy being a source of useful work. Tiller took an engineering pathway and consciously moved toward building the bridge in terms of the physical sciences, of joining "the inner" and "the outer," connecting well-known principles of heat and work. As a theoretical physicist, his main thrust was that the hypothesis must be empirically testable and falsifiable. Critics of Tiller's method may declare we cannot bring intention and put it in a flask in the lab, that intention is not subject to being tested via the physical sciences.

This leads to the discussion of the nature of science itself. Paradoxically, science is a verb, not a noun. Science is an activity, a means of inquiry, and not just a collection of subjects like physics or biology.[112] Science as an activity also means it is an inquiry into what it means to have an intention. Tiller looked at the overall scheme and defined the problem: Consciousness does things by intention, and consciousness is the human connection to Spirit. You cannot provide proof of these statements. Regard them instead as self-evident. As Tiller sees it, you have to start somewhere. You have to make an assumption and explore consequences.

Tiller says: "Scientific tools and our ability to discriminate say something about our degree of evolution. How finely can you distinguish between states in Nature? In the Upanishads, there are fifteen variations of the unconscious state. The sages who wrote the Upanishads had advanced abilities to differentiate and, therefore, could have more states. Truth depends on how finely the information is described."

In Tiller's mind, the question isn't "Am I capable?" The question is "What should I build?" Tiller has the inner game, the right stuff, *adaequatio*. Framed properly and understood properly, Tiller takes the angle of consciousness performing useful work. And work means consciousness via intention must be a source of energy. Using this schema, Tiller taught me something much larger than physics. He taught me about a particular type of imagination, both unique and pragmatic, that amounted to a form of genius, a type of genius that engineered a link, and in a flash, conceived of a way forward in bridge building. Work and energy point to fundamental laws in physics, which form a mighty pillar in all of science. We come to this junction of the bridge in the next pillar.

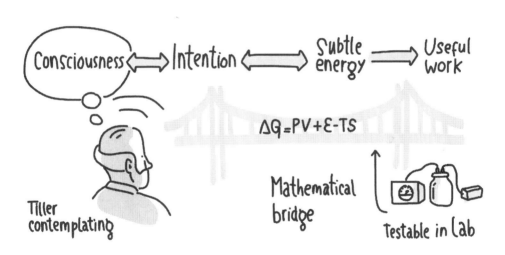

Every bridge is a storyteller, telling the story of a particular place and the technology of its time. Since a bridge is always experienced in its totality, its design is inextricable from its location, which encompasses geological conditions, traffic patterns, and the natural and built environment.

—Judith Dupre

Bridges: A History of the World's Most Spectacular Spans[113]

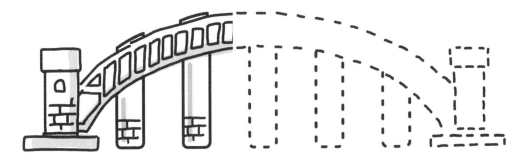

BRIDGE PILLAR 3:
Of the Mighty Second Law of Thermodynamics, Entropy, and Information

A good many times I have been present at gatherings of people who, by the standards of the traditional culture, are thought highly educated and who have with considerable gusto been expressing their incredulity at the illiteracy of scientists. Once or twice I have been provoked and have asked the company how many of them could describe the Second Law of Thermodynamics. The response was cold; it was also negative. Yet I was asking something which is about the scientific equivalent of: *Have you read a work of Shakespeare's?*

–C. P. SNOW, *The Two Cultures and the Scientific Revolution*[114]

A theory is the more impressive the greater the simplicity of its premises, the more different kinds of things it relates, and the more extended its area of applicability. Therefore, the deep impression that classical thermodynamics made upon me. It is the only physical theory of universal content which I am convinced will never be overthrown, within the framework of applicability of its basic concepts.

–ALBERT EINSTEIN[115]

We have developed these mathematical laws based
ultimately on a set of definitions of mass, charge, space, and time.
We don't really know what these quantities are,
but we have defined them to have certain unchanging properties
and have thus constructed our edifice of knowledge on these pillars.
The edifice will be stable so long as the pillars are unchanging.

–WILLIAM A. TILLER[116]

[15]
"Learn thermodynamics.
The terms of the second law hold the keys
to understanding nature."
The Universal Laws of Thermodynamics

In my third Thursday meeting with Tiller, he laid a critical pillar for the bridge. Writing in his characteristic large, capitalized scrawl, he outlined the laws of thermodynamics on a piece of paper.

Among the hundreds of physical laws that describe the universe, the laws of thermodynamics are mighty. In science, the word "law" is significant. "Law" means it holds in all places and all times. Like a Shakespearean drama, the story of thermodynamics in the mid-1800s involves powerful and finely drawn characters. Thermodynamics isn't only about heat and work; it has fundamental implications for human life. Scientists trust these laws more than any other.

Beneath the equations on my piece of paper are real-world applications. Processes such as a car rolling down a hill, a cup of hot coffee cooling down, modern refrigeration, and the muscles in my hand as I type these words—all look different. Yet they are all driven by the laws of thermodynamics. Having read more than thirty-five physics textbooks since that fateful Thursday meeting, I will not provide a "how to" but rather a "what it's all about" of the underlying principles.

In his brilliant book *Understanding Thermodynamics,*[117] chemical engineer Hendrick Van Ness summarized the first law of thermodynamics: Energy is conserved. Any conservation law involves *accounting.* We know there is a fixed amount of something, and we need merely find the various pieces that add up to, or account for, the total. We hold this law to be implicit for all situations. That's just another way of saying that we believe in the first law.

As Van Ness writes: Why do we believe in it? Certainly, no one has proved it. On the other hand, no one has been able to find anything wrong with it. All we know is that it has worked in every instance where it has been applied, and we are happy with it simply because it works. Why does it work? We haven't the faintest idea; it's just a miracle of nature. The conservation law is a *description* of how nature works, not an explanation. Fortunately, that's all we need. Although we do not know why it works, we do know how it works.

The second law had a humble beginning with the observation that heat does not spontaneously flow from a cold object to a hotter object. Everyday experience tells us that certain processes occur spontaneously, and certain processes do not. Hot coffee loses heat to the surrounding air until both reach the same temperature—a state of thermal equilibrium, and there is no further heat exchanged. Energy is conserved in this process. The word "equilibrium" implies a state of balance; there are no unbalanced potentials or forces (in our case, temperature differences) in the system. Another way to look at it is that equilibrium is the most *probable* state. The coffee doesn't suddenly extract more heat from the air, making itself hotter and the air even cooler. Experience tells us this doesn't happen.

Now, if you take the mechanical process of a car rolling down a hill, it is distinctly different from the hot coffee as a thermal process. Yet it is intriguing that we can say similar things about both processes. In each case, we readily see the cause of the process and can correctly predict the changes that will occur. In other words, we can see the "direction" of each process.

In our meeting, Tiller wrote a version of the second law known as the Gibbs free energy equation. In the Gibbs free energy equation, *(G)* equals pressure times volume *(PV)* plus internal energy *(E)* minus temperature times entropy *(TS)*:

$$G = PV + E - TS$$

While sipping our hot coffee, we contemplate these terms. If we "captured" the heat flow process from the hot coffee to the cooler air, we might harness that heat energy for useful work. Although this seems far-fetched, in fact, from this very nitty-gritty beginning, French physicist Nicolas Léonard Sadi Carnot deduced a practical way to capture heat for work, thereby laying the foundations of thermodynamics in 1824. In the case of our coffee cooling spontaneously, this is where the word "free" comes from: It refers to the amount of energy in a system that is readily available for usage. Heated water and steam expand in the closed volume of a boiler. The pressure of the steam is powerful enough to drive an engine, so long as enough heat is continually supplied to the water keep it in a state of steam. Pressure times volume *(PV)* is fundamental to the "age of steam." The *PV* term leads to a positive change in Gibbs free energy, or ΔG for short. The symbol "Δ" means "change in."

Still sipping our coffee, we note the internal energy term denoted by *E*. This looks familiar, and it is. It is the famous *E* in $E = mc^2$. We note that mass *(m)* and energy *(E)* are on equal footing thanks to Einstein's insight. This mass–energy relationship is a basis for nuclear atomic power. Einstein's equation revealed that mass itself (or matter) has an associated energy that can be released if the matter is destroyed. Think of the massive and sudden ΔG released from nuclear fission that can destroy entire cities. We gulp our coffee. As we do so, we note that this internal energy is known only as a function of other things. We cannot measure or define it. We have merely an equation that tells us how to measure its change.

Our coffee nearly cold and almost gone, we notice that T stands for temperature. Temperature is typically used to signify how hot something is. In a moment of *eureka!* we realize something more profound and fundamental about temperature. When we measure the temperature of our coffee, we are recording the average energy or motion of the particles that make it up. Temperature is related to the average speed at which the particles vibrate and bounce around. It's a macroscopic description of the kinetic energy of a group of particles. Thus, technically, temperature is an energy unit. Because it is clumsy to talk about temperature in terms of the unit of energy, joules, we stick with the familiar degrees: Celsius, Fahrenheit, or Kelvin.

An implication of the second law is that converting heat to energy to do work is not perfect. In any process that changes heat into another form of energy, a little energy is wasted. Carnot, in his book *Reflections on the Motive Power of Fire,* expressed his theory of maximum efficiency of heat engines. Using Carnot's knowledge, the austere physicist Rudolph Clausius set down the second law of thermodynamics in the form "heat cannot of itself pass from one body to a hotter body."

From this experimental generalization, Clausius deduced that it was impossible to neatly transform all the heat into work. In seeking a formal measure of the energy *not* transformed into work, Clausius, in 1865, introduced the German word *entropie,* derived from the Greek root *tropie,* or "transformation."[118] Entropy, denoted by S, helps us determine the amount of energy that cannot be recovered or is unavailable to do work. Simply put, entropy is a loss of energy, an increase in disorder. The minus sign before *TS* signifies energy that is not transferred. So, entropy is a negative kind of quantity, the opposite of available energy.

Temperature is directly related to entropy; cold bodies have low entropy. Their atoms are less disordered than those in hot bodies, which jiggle around more. As our hot coffee cools, its molecules lose energy and became more "ordered." If we continue cooling the coffee (in the freezer), the result, iced coffee, would have molecules that are much more ordered and maybe even more delicious. In the cooling process, energy is transferred to the air, which becomes warmer and more disordered.

"Disorder" is a central idea of the second law and one that I will use in this book to mean the opposite of organization or order. This kind of entropy is commonly understood as thermodynamic entropy. The qualifier "thermodynamic" is necessary because the word entropy is also used in other, non-thermodynamic ideas, such as spreading and information.

It is sort of intuitive that entropy and temperature play a role describing the "spontaneous" part of the process. A high temperature implies that molecules are bouncing around and more likely to change their arrangement. Furthermore, an increase in entropy usually means the system has moved to a "more probable," that is, more likely state.

We can now look for an easily understood statement that provides an obvious answer to the question: "Is a process spontaneous or not?" It boils down to Gibbs free energy. Tiller advised me: "Always go back to ΔG. In short, excess free energy drives the universe. Changes in any of the terms—ΔP, ΔV, ΔE, ΔT, and ΔS, or combinations thereof—can lead to available free energy for useful work. Your consciousness can be a source of excess free energy, too. Always go back to ΔG. That's the important part."

How can consciousness be a source of Gibbs free energy? This is moonshot kind of thinking.

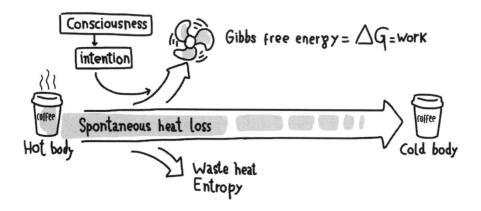

[16]
"Boltzmann bridged the macroscopic world you see and observe with the microscopic world of atoms."
A Tortured Mind: Ludwig Boltzmann (1844–1906)

On a Thursday morning, I am preparing green tea for Tiller and myself. The jasmine aroma molecules from the unfurling tea leaves don't stay sequestered in the teapot. Instead, the jasmine fragrance quickly disperses throughout my kitchen and into the apartment, then spreads to the apartment next door, tickling my neighbor's nostrils, then bouncing and jostling freely down the road. Soon, jasmine molecules spread throughout Scottsdale and eventually circle the entire Earth, reaching equilibrium. Maybe you're breathing in one of those wayward molecules right now.

Suppose the windows and door of my apartment are kept shut. Would the jasmine molecules inside my apartment ever return to the pot? What are the chances of that happening? Most will say it's impossible. Austrian physicist Ludwig Boltzmann would say: "Well, there may be a tiny probability that one day, who knows how long from now, all of the molecules will find their way back."[119]

The magic word: *probability*.[120] It is exceedingly probable for the jasmine molecules to disperse rather than stay bunched up in one place. Probability dictates what we observe. As time passes, molecules become more and more mixed. Cold and hot liquids in contact with each other equalize into lukewarm. An ink swirl in water disperses to a pale blue color. Nature moves, always, spontaneously in the direction of increasing entropy until it reaches equilibrium or maximum spread. Therefore, equilibrium is the highest level of entropy.

Ludwig Boltzmann formulated these ideas in 1879. There is a finite probability— vanishingly small, in this case—that molecules will one day return, that the teapot will once again have an intense perfume of jasmine. We can understand many things about matter by understanding it as consisting of tiny identical components like atoms and molecules in some state of motion.

Boltzmann was not unknown to me when Tiller first mentioned his name. But as often is the case in the sciences, his name had previously appeared in an equation, utterly impersonal. The full import eluded me until I read about his life and tragic end. In the late nineteenth century, atoms were not an accepted part of physics. After all, equations described heat and work correctly, and the matter was considered closed. Besides, no one had seen any atoms. Who, then, in God's name could support such ghostly entities? Atoms? Totally ridiculous.

Boltzmann, however, championed the idea of atoms. Whereas others saw steam as a gas and nothing else, Boltzmann saw molecules moving in a frenzy, pushing on each other and on the container, creating pressure. The frenzied state was the most probable state: entropy. We measure the average qualities of all the billions of molecules and arrive at macroscopic properties we can measure: temperature, pressure, and work.

These are the properties that interest us. We could care less about the motions of every molecule in the system. Boltzmann provided a way, one of the most powerful methods in thermal physics, to predict the macroscopic properties of systems by averaging all possible solutions of the mechanical system at the atomic level. The second law of thermodynamics is a probabilistic law.

Over shouting matches at scientific conferences in Vienna, Boltzmann endured harsh criticism and fierce opposition to his theory of atomism. His moods see-sawed along with his theory's rejection and occasional acceptance.[121]

Tormented by depression and fear of lecturing, Boltzmann confronted his scientific isolation. In one of his opening lectures, we sense his delicate nature as he addressed his students: "Forgive me if I have not accomplished much. . . . I only wanted to offer you something quite modest. But forgive me, if before we go on, I ask you for something that is most important to me: your confidence, your sympathy, your love, in a word the greatest thing you are able to give, yourself."[122]

In 1906, at the age of sixty-two, Boltzmann's will ran out. While on summer holiday in Duino, on the shores of the Adriatic near Trieste, this great physicist took his own life. Alas, he acted too hastily, for a few years later his theories were completely triumphant. In 1913 Jean Baptiste Perrin published his classic book on atomic theory, *Les Atomes*.[123] A great deal of modern chemical science emerged from the firm foundations established in *Les Atomes*. By 1926, the Perrin-Boltzmann message had been so successful that no one doubted the atomic hypotheses.

The famous Boltzmann equation is $S = k \log(W)$. Here S is the thermodynamic entropy and W represents the number of ways the individual microscopic molecules (such as a gas or jasmine molecules) can arrange themselves. If we consider the teapot, there are many ways the jasmine molecules can disperse. Therefore, W is a huge number. This equation tells us that we do not need to know what every molecule in our teapot is doing. The Boltzmann constant, k, is a conversion factor relating energy at the individual molecule level to its temperature. Boltzmann's constant is a truly small number to balance out the huge W, a bridge between microscopic and macroscopic worlds. If we know some of the factors affecting *W*, such as the number of molecules or the change in volume, then we can calculate the entropy of the system. The number of molecules could be a dozen or a standard mole (6.022×10^{23} molecules). The logarithm function allows for simpler calculations for huge numbers.

Regarding my example of the system of high entropy and disorder with the jasmine molecules, my knowledge of the overall macroscopic state of the system (teapot and apartment) tells me very little about which of the possible microstates it is in. The individual behavior of each jasmine molecule is hard to predict. Importantly, I am ignorant of and cannot distinguish one configuration of the molecules from another. Entropy is then proportional to my ignorance and lack of information about the microstates. Boltzmann's foremost success came in an 1878 paper showing that systems composed of many particles tended toward states that had as little information as possible.

It seems to me that Boltzmann's equation speaks to life itself, which, in my case, resembles a jumble. Tracing my path would look like one of those gas atoms that Boltzmann described. Zig here, zag there. Dizzying progress as my (blood) pressure rises, then frustratingly slow, and speeding up again . . . The arrow of time moving forward.

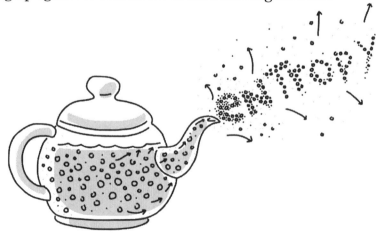

[17]
"Thermodynamics is essential to biology."
Spread Your Power: Disequilibrium Thermodynamics

Enjoying the warm sunshine in Scottsdale, I cannot help but marvel at the giant thermonuclear battery in the sky. The thermodynamic machinery starts with solar radiation spreading through a hierarchy of levels, a trophic pyramid of power.[124] As long as there is an energy gradient, energy flows from a high level to low, doing work. The energy difference or "disequilibrium" powers all processes: Winds blow, rivers flow, the mantle convects, continents drift, and life grows. The Earth is in a state of constant disequilibrium.

Photosynthesis harnesses the free energy of sunlight and converts it to chemical free energy by splitting water and carbon dioxide. Thus, photosynthesis transfers power to the rest of the biosphere, including us. Boltzmann was the first scientist to note the role of photosynthesis in decreasing entropy and bringing order to living matter.

To envision thermodynamics and life in proper perspective, we start with the time-honored view of biology as unity within diversity.[125] Unity emerges when we penetrate beneath the surface to the intracellular machinery and processes by which species grow and reproduce. Examination at the microscopic level reveals common features of cell and organelle structure. Continuing down the size range, we come to biochemistry, a collection of thousands of enzymatic reactions by which a cell shapes matter and energy into forms appropriate for its own purposes.

Here the full impact of thermodynamics is evident, for almost every sequence of biochemistry involves reactions with molecules of adenosine triphosphate. These reactions apply to all the millions of species that inhabit Earth. This ubiquitous molecule, best known by the abbreviation ATP, is central to energy processing in all cells. ATP is the final energy transfer molecule in almost all cellular processes. Muscles, fireflies, and electric eels are all powered by energy temporarily stored in ATP. In animal cells, almost all of the energy used for ATP synthesis comes from the oxidation of sugars.

Zooming in to the interior of our cells, driving them, providing the oxidative energy that sends us out for improvement each shining day, are the mitochondria. Without them, we would not move a muscle, drum a finger, or think a thought.[126] Protein molecules embedded in the mitochondrial membrane pump protons and ions from one side of the membrane to the other. Energy is thereby stored in the form of a charge separation and coupled to ATP production. These tiny ionic cell factories convert chemical energy into mechanical work with almost 100 percent efficiency.

In addition to the chemical potentials, there are many other potentials, such as kinetic, rotational, internal energy aspects, and so on. The total energy, ΔG, is determined by the sum total, or accounting, of the various contributions driving cellular processes. It isn't energy per se, but rather the flow of energy through a system, that does work and acts to organize that system.[127] Coupled with energy flow, our cells manage not to fall apart because they continually increase the entropy around them to increase the order within them. Their molecular structure lets them absorb energy to perform work and release heat.

This ability to absorb energy allows our cells to refine their structure, create furnaces like the mitochondria, absorb more energy to do more work, and, in the process, dissipate more heat. It all adds up to a positive feedback loop. In this process, the energy remains the same and external entropy increases. It is entropy that cannot be turned back. The second law of thermodynamics demands it. What makes the world go round are not sources of energy but sources of low entropy.

Central to biological order, life needs nonequilibrium thermo-dynamics. If all temperature gradient inequalities were eliminated, intelligent life on Earth would not be possible. Take in energy and dissipate it as heat; that's the most essential process.

Thermodynamics = you.

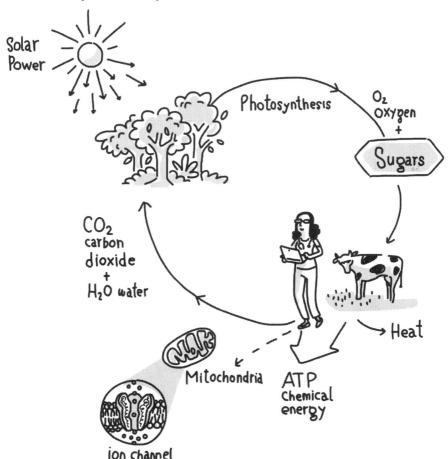

[18]
"People say that life violates the second law of thermodynamics. This is not the case; we know of nothing in the universe that violates that law."
Simulations and Stimulations: From Soup to Solid State

A tree and a solar panel both absorb and transform solar energy and release heat into their environment. How would a physicist explain why only the tree is alive? We think we know life when we see it. But what is the difference between a rooster and a rock, when both obey the same physical laws? In other words, how do you say "life" in physics?[128]

If thermodynamics encompasses the laws of nature, then maybe it can tell us about the conditions of the very beginning of life. We are going back billions of years to the primordial soup. Was life just a lucky chance? Like fifty-fifty? Was it one in a trillion? We are back to the question of probabilities of living things, which, at the most basic level, take in energy and throw out waste heat. How did atoms and molecules, the building blocks of matter, organize themselves in the primordial soup to become more lifelike? Can thermodynamics tell us when and under what conditions lifelike behaviors emerged?

Suppose you take a crucible and put in ingredients essential for life: water, carbon, nitrogen, phosphorus, sulfur. How does physical order resembling life emerge from such a primordial soup? Nobel Laureate chemist Ilya Prigogine had similarly wondered why order arises spontaneously in nature.[129] How does water vapor reorganize and cascade down as perfect six-sided snowflakes, each different, each detailed as though God himself fashioned it? How does physical order emerge from a system that does not have any patterns—or, in other words, organization—of atoms and molecules, from amorphous water vapor into a perfect six-sided crystal with sixty-degree angles?

Thermodynamics may hold important answers. Nonequilibrium thermodynamics is a relatively new and hot field of physics. "Nonequilibrium" means a system, such as our primordial soup, is kept in a constant, perturbed state, like continually flicking your little sibling in the ear.

We know that ΔG drives all processes. Energy equals work. We also know the most probable state for life is taking in energy so that atoms or molecules can do work and throw off heat, or entropy, to their surroundings. Entropy is the essential key to life. While at University of California, Berkeley, chemist Gavin Crooks wrote an equation showing that the crucial means for a system to organize is throwing off heat energy, a process called "dissipation." Dissipation further results in a process that goes forward, along the "arrow of time."[130] Heat and time are bound together in an intricate dance, and the dissipation of heat is what stops time from going backward. Heat energy becomes not only unavailable but irrecoverable in any form. Crooks was able to prove mathematically that in a quantitative sense, the dissipation of heat—entropy—is the price we pay for the arrow of time. The more a system increases the entropy of its surroundings, the less reversible it becomes.

Taking the crucible of primordial soup, you zap it with a good jolt of electricity. You keep disturbing the soup by putting in work (energy) with an electromagnetic field. Instead of only increasing the kinetic energy of disorganized movement (temperature) as we are used to, it also causes irreversible self-organizing changes.

Just such a transformation has been created in simulations by physicist Jeremy England of the Massachusetts Institute of Technology (MIT).[131] By asking how a system far from equilibrium (having a large gradient) manages to keep itself from running down to equilibrium, England has shown in computer simulations that the primordial soup's entropy production is critical. Amazingly, atoms organize into molecules, which in turn organize themselves into structures that take in energy and dissipate it as heat. When England tweaks the formula of energy input, the molecular organization changes accordingly. Evidently, a little bubbling, whirling, and seething goes a long way in organizing matter. This understanding has led to the birth of a new science. It seems that the probability of lifelike self-organizing stuff in the lab is possible.[132]

A soup of common materials, even if self-organizing, is all well and good, but something is still missing. The self-organizing dissipating semisolid soup cannot talk, love, complain, create, or read this fascinating chapter, and do all the things that constitute our humanity. How do we assemble the self-organizing thingamajig into cells, cells into tissues, tissues into organs, and organs into a person? It staggers the imagination.

The key point is that, although the second law is necessary for the emergence of complex order, it is far from sufficient. Life is inherently an out-of-equilibrium phenomenon, but then so is an explosion. Something other than nonequilibrium thermodynamics is needed to explain why life and explosions are fundamentally different.

Thermodynamics takes us impressively forward. But we come to a halt. The scientific reasons become clearer. Energy is needed for information to emerge. We are, at the molecular level, the most information-dense structures around, squirming with information at every covalent bond, surpassing by magnitudes the best that computer engineers can design. Information is a crucial brick for the bridge.

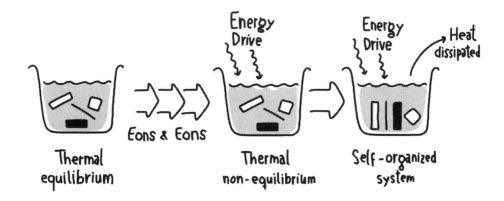

[19]
"The most fundamental aspect of the universe and reality is information. It's more fundamental than matter or energy. Information is the gateway and bridge to understanding ourselves."
A Playful Mind: Claude Elwood Shannon (1916–2001)

We have looked at thermodynamics: heat and work, probabilities and entropy, biology and energy gradients, far-from-equilibrium systems, and dissipative systems that mimic primitive lifelike organizations. There is an even more impressive and unifying principle underlying all these concepts. Far more powerful than energy or matter, it speaks to the deep analogies between very different extremes of physics and between physics and life. It is information.

In everyday parlance, information is frequently synonymous with knowledge. The first definition of information in Merriam-Webster's dictionary reflects this idea: Information is "the communication or reception of knowledge or intelligence." To understand the power of information, we owe much to the genius and playful mind of Claude Shannon. A juggler, unicyclist, chess player, and even a blackjack gambler, Shannon joined his engineering background with mathematics for the rarest of insights into communication between humans: Communication can be measured with units, just like measuring the temperature or weight of something. By doing so, he launched the digital information age.

In 1948, Shannon posed a question: How much does it cost to transmit messages from one place to another? He worked at Bell Laboratories, AT&T's famous research unit. He was studying the difficulty of transmitting messages using electromagnetic signals down a telephone line. Say you want to send a message to your mom across the pond. When sending the message "I love you," you'd want to be sure it is encoded properly by the electromagnetic wires, transmitted without static, and received error-free on the other side of the Atlantic. To Shannon's engineering mind, the meaning of a message was irrelevant to his question. For "I love you" or "I hate you," you'd get the same bill from AT&T for your call. AT&T doesn't care what you say, in English, Kiswahili, or Gujarati; your bill reflects the length of the call.

Shannon's analysis converted information, not as a psychological thing, but as a physical one. Shannon insisted that meaning had nothing to do with information. This was critical. He was concerned with how to protect a message from the power lines, heat, and noise; a problem he tackled with engineering precision. The strategy Shannon used to create his information units was to ask how frequently letters and their arrangement are used, for example, in English.

For simplification, there are twenty-six individual letters, but letters are not used equally. Vowels and letters like *t, s,* and *h* are used more frequently than is the letter *z*. Crossword puzzle devotees and Scrabble players know this. A rare letter narrows the choice of words far more than a common letter and conveys more information to solve the clues about an incomplete word.[133] Each letter has a probability distribution proportional to its frequency of use and, consequently, its information measure. Likewise, certain words are more probable from all the millions of letter arrangements.

Next, if we want to compress and squeeze a string of characters, the probabilities become key to the engineering task. Shannon was concerned with communicating the microstate of a system, such as the arrangement of letters. He equated information with entropy.

Shannon bumped into the same principle as Boltzmann: probability. Boltzmann was describing all the countless probable arrangements of gas molecules of a system so we can "see" how the whole behaves.

In the analogous information function, Shannon was describing all the countless probable arrangements of the letters of the alphabet to see how they transmit communication. In Boltzmann's formula, entropy refers to an average of physical states (such as temperature), and in Shannon's formula, information refers to a particular physical state (such as the specific sentence, "I love you.").[134] The fact that Boltzmann and Shannon both derived the same equation points to the deeply physical nature of information.

Shannon's theory is more general than is Boltzmann's because it applies to any kind of aggregates or physical order. Think of geneticists and the information contained in DNA or about the information contained in an opera score, a reel of film, or this book. In these examples, the word *information* refers to the presence of order. Shannon's theory applies to any linear array of order in symbols, which may be letters, musical notes, experimental observations, amino acids in a linear peptide, or any other defined sequence.

Shannon's work led to the 1948 publication of his famous paper "A Mathematical Theory of Communication."[135] In this landmark paper, he described a measure—the minimum value—required to uniquely specify a message. His measure was based on the binary digit, either zero or a one, and was called a "bit." A series of binary choices—on/off, true/false, 1/0—was Shannon's first great feat of abstraction. Information comes in discrete units, one bit at a time. We cannot divide this bit into smaller units. However, you can compress this sentence using a string of bits, such as "0000111010101," transmit it down a line with less heat and less signal loss, and then decode the bits at the receiving end. More than that, you can compress a whole lot of messages to bits, allowing your telephone line to transmit a lot more communication; in other words, increasing its bandwidth. More bandwidth, more bits per second, means more revenue for AT&T.

At least in the simplest cases, Shannon said, the information content of a message was the number of binary ones and zeroes required to encode it. If you knew in advance that a message would convey a simple choice—yes or no, true or false—then one binary digit would suffice. A single zero or a single one would tell you all you needed to know. The message would thus be defined to have one unit of information. A more complicated message, on the other hand, would require more digits to encode and would contain that much more information. Think of the thousands or millions of ones and zeroes that make up a word processing file.[136]

Shannon's momentous question—How much does it cost to communicate?—showed that information, rather than being an abstract notion, is entirely a physical quantity. In this sense, it is at least on an equal footing with energy and work. Now we have brought information up to the important level of energy and matter.

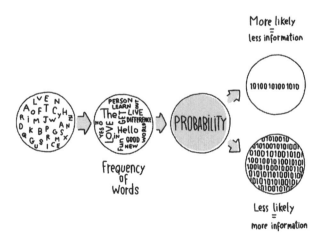

[20]
"Information is related to entropy."
The Negentropy Principle of Information[137]

In 1929, the Hungarian physicist Leo Szilard posed an excellent question: Can you know about the world without changing it? The answer was simple: No, you cannot.[138] Shannon asked what it costs to transmit knowledge. Szilard asked how much it costs to measure, to attain knowledge. With this question, Szilard launched the study of gaining knowledge in the physical world: measurement as a material act, knowing as work, sensation as metabolism, thought as thermodynamics. This is significant in the history of human knowledge.

To know, we must make observations, or measurements, of materials and the environment. We require some physical indicator to detect or see the molecules or images or anything else. Such indicators require an expenditure of energy. The physicist in his laboratory needs a power supply: batteries, compressed gases, and so on. He also needs light to read gauges, meters, and instruments.

Knowledge costs. In his 1956 book *Science and Information Theory*, French physicist Léon Brillouin showed that this aforementioned laboratory power expenditure leads to as much molecular disordering in the measurements: Entropy increases somewhere in the system.[139] The crux of this scientific argument is that you cannot get something for nothing, not even information. Energy must be expended in learning about the state of a system, and *gaining* information *increases* entropy.

If we consider Boltzmann's statistical mechanics, entropy is usually described as measuring the amount of disorder in a physical system. This viewpoint takes into account that we, as observers of the system, do not have information, or are ignorant of the exact micro-state the system is in. More precisely, entropy is a measure of our lack of information because in practice we are unable to distinguish a great variety of microscopically distinct states from one another. The question then arises: Is entropy a property of the system, of the observer, or of the relationship between them?[140] The second law of thermodynamics and entropy tell us as much about the observer as about the system.

The relationship between entropy and information within a system can be illustrated with my teapot and jasmine molecule example. Consider the small chamber of the teapot and large chamber of the kitchen. A molecule is in one of the two chambers, but we do not know which one. In general, as a jasmine molecule goes from a state of lower entropy (in teapot) to a state of higher entropy (kitchen space), we go from a state of lower uncertainty about its location (somewhere within the few cubic inches of the teapot) to a state of greater uncertainty (somewhere within a few cubic yards of the kitchen).

The amount of certainty or information we have in determining a jasmine molecule's location corresponds to its entropy level, with less uncertainty corresponding to lower entropy. When we are more certain of the state of the jasmine molecule, we have gained real information. Therefore, reduction in uncertainty represents an increase in information; that is, a decrease of entropy corresponds to an increase in our actual knowledge about a jasmine molecule. Brillouin established a new term for negative entropy, "negentropy." So, negentropy is information. The key point to remember is that *entropy is proportional to* a function that measures *our lack of information about the microstate of a system.*[141]

Brillouin based his calculations on physical measurements. But he failed to ask if a scientist can *feel* his way around. In plain old-fashioned physics, intention or feeling does not counter the laws of thermodynamics, as we shall see. This introduces a subtle point, since there is the possibility that you as the observer and the system will, in fact, be one thing.[142] The boundaries of any system are, in a sense, arbitrary and nonexistent. The observer is always inextricably linked to the system.

Shannon was interested in the amount of data in each message, but not in the meaning and relevance, which are vital to the question of consciousness. There must be something else present, something more than words. After all, children learn from observing the grownups around them. They do this over and over again. They learn from narratives and fairy tales and on the playground. A little girl takes a jumbled pile of Play-Doh and creates a ball, an orderly shape. She grows up and sees a jumbled heap of sand, and with information in her mind, creates a ball of glass, five centimeters across. Her intention is made physical, and we can say something about it in informational terms, such as its dimensions and material properties. By shaping the chaotic sand into a glass ball, information is rendered into a physical thing that endures. We are back to intention, back to ourselves as creators. We create order, we create negentropy with information.

Tiller often says: "The second law has terms that can be discriminated by today's scientific tools: pressure, volume, internal energy, temperature, and entropy. An intention, human emotions, the mind, all can also set up [as a source of] Gibb's free energy. In future, we will have the tools to discriminate the contributions, that is, ΔG of the mind, ΔG of emotion, ΔG of consciousness, ΔG of intention. Human intention and emotion would be treated as information and beyond

Shannon 'bits.' We don't see all the variables and cannot yet describe the science. As such, it's all an approximation of the truth."

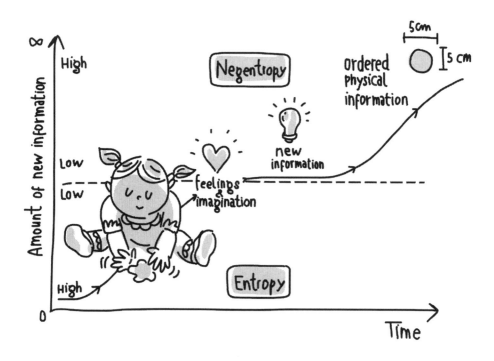

[21]
"Entropy and information are crucial to biology."
Entropy and Your Diet

The connection between entropy, energy, and information reveals something of its usefulness in daily life. Energy concerns us especially with its connection to body weight. Entropy concerns us with its connection to our physical deterioration. In his influential 1944 monograph *What Is Life?*, the eminent quantum physicist Erwin Schrödinger suggested that in addition to displaying the energy content of food (calories), its negative entropy potential—the degree to which the composition of the food allows us to combat entropy—should also be displayed.[143]

Interestingly, Schrödinger used the term "negative entropy," but he was criticized for using it because technically the food does not provide negative entropy itself but the "free energy" used to achieve a state of order. He, in turn, argued that his book was for the layperson and that "free energy" would be confused with "energy." For our discussion, I will use "entropy" as additional information on food packaging.

Imagine you're in your local supermarket in the sweet's aisle. The chocolate bar you're eyeing shows you an energy amount on its wrapper in kilocalories: 250 kcal or joules. That's the amount of heat your body will generate if you eat the whole thing. Sure, there will be intermediary steps in biochemistry, such as forming covalent bonds and such, but for purposes of discussion of entropy and your diet, we can skip over these aspects to the essential point.

Suppose that in addition to the energy content, the chocolate bar's label also displayed its entropy potential, telling you that eating this bar would contribute ten units of entropy. The label could say something like: "Entropy: 10 units, sucrose and theobromine." It would mean that eating the chocolate bar will supply your mitochondrial factories with materials to make lots of energy in the form of ATP. However, in addition to energy, your cells also need diverse molecular information—not just that contained in the sugar (sucrose) and cocoa (alkaloid theobromine), but also in trace minerals and vitamins. Put another way, you could eat chocolate bars for breakfast, lunch, and dinner, but you'd be missing crucial nutritional information required to keep your body in a highly ordered or low entropy state.[144]

You head to the fresh produce aisle. Maybe an all-grapefruit diet is a better option. It's healthier, right? Your meal plan is to eat fresh grapefruit for breakfast, broiled grapefruit for lunch, and juiced grapefruit for dinner. It has plenty of water, vitamin C, potassium, and fiber, and provides energy as fructose. Yet the outcome of the grapefruit diet is that it, too, is missing crucial information to keep your body in an ordered state. Pretty soon into the grapefruit phase, aside from getting indigestion, your body degenerates into a disordered state and, worse, may become dysfunctional. Alas, another diet bites the dust.

All this suggests the best foods are those that give a specified high energy value with the lowest entropy increase in the body. Food's entropy value is correlated to its completeness, in terms of the range of nutrients, as well as the bioavailability of the nutrients. This is the concept of a balanced diet.[145] Of course, high-entropy foods can be combined with other foods and nutrients to reduce the overall entropy contribution to your body.

Eating chocolate as I wrote this section, I had a sudden ah-ha moment that information is more than the nutrients contained in my confection. The sheen and gloss of my chocolate gave me information about its freshness and quality, confirmed by the sharp snap as I broke off a piece, setting free odor molecules that added a tiny, distinctive chemical signature to the air, providing more information about what's in my chocolate. The miniature chemistry lab of sensing cells deep inside my nose decoded the chemical messages, creating a unique pattern I interpret as the aroma of great chocolate. Information in sight, sound, and smell.

Food for thought.

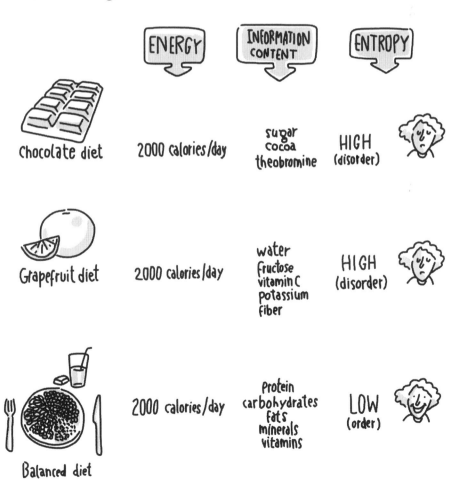

The unassuming poetry of bridges reveals itself to those who would see it. Whether a simple or more complex crossing, each of these structures has much to say about the extraordinary lives, effort, ingenuity, and wonder that come together on a bridge.

—Judith Dupre

Bridges: A History of the World's Most Spectacular Spans.[146]

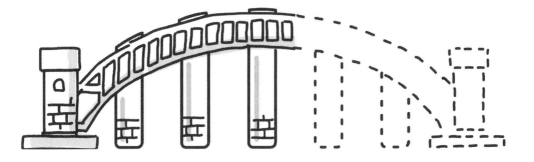

BRIDGE PILLAR 4:
Four Target Experiments That Bridge Human Intention to Physical Reality in the Laboratory

*Verily, verily, I say unto you, He that believeth on me,
the works that I do shall he do also; and greater works than these
shall he do; because I go unto my Father.*

–JOHN 14:12

"Miracles" don't necessarily defy the laws of nature.
They're a bit less grandiose than that—instead, a miracle is a
phenomenon that was previously considered unimaginable.
Witnesses to that miracle are called upon to reframe their
assumptions and resolve contradictions. In short, they must
start to think about their world in a new light.

–WILLIAM A. TILLER[147]

[22]
"Intention is a process of creation."
A Radically Subjective "Inside-Out" Science

We come to the central section of the bridge. In pillar four, we test the design and functionality of Tiller's hypothesis by experiment and find out if his novel science protocol can bridge great gaps in consciousness research. The details of his protocol's construction emerge from distinct yet interdependent conditions: context, design, and connection. I include this essay because it is easy to gloss over a critical preparatory phase in the intention experimental protocol: the powerful intention statement. The context had constraints: a limited budget from private funding only, and the challenge of performing a test on intention, a test having little scientific precedent in a world of MRI brain science. The protocol, if successful, would provide the data to close the gap between intention and its material physical outcomes.

Tiller selected the first target material to test his intention: water. If there is "magic" on this planet, it is contained in water.[148] A water molecule is made up of two hydrogen atoms and one oxygen atom. The representation of water as H_2O, based on this fact, is part of our common folk knowledge.

Tiller expressed his intention using his creative tool: the written word. And like a sculptor, language is his scalpel, his scientific hammer and chisel. He created information with words and equations, not in a string of Shannon-like bits of zeroes and ones. Tiller refined his process using his well-worn spiralbound notebook and his favorite pen.

Using water as an example, his protocol involves:

- Seeing the three-dimensional structural arrangement of H_2O's atoms in relation to each other, using his materials science mind.[149] He takes in the structure of water and its possibilities. The clue to some of water's strange behavior resides in the weak hydrogen bonds and the van der Waals bonds between water molecules. Liquid water is so intricately interlaced that it is almost a continuous structure, and a glass of water can be thought of as one giant molecule. This range of weak bonds gives water both extraordinary strength and astonishing flexibility.

• Visualizing water, contemplating it, in his imagination—this way, that way, jotting in his notebook. The glass of water serenely sitting on his desk consists of 10^{24} molecules, which are constantly moving about, dissociating into hydrogen and hydroxyl ions and then re-associating, forming and unforming microcrystals, and colliding with the walls of the container. Because individual molecules are so small, we only see averages over vast numbers of particles, hence the illusion of great regularity.

• Writing equations to give mathematical expression to changes in water. Words are interspersed among them, like stamps of approval. "Under standard conditions, of ambient temperature and pressure, the K_w constant shows the self-ionization of water, the ion product: $K_w = [H3O+][HO-] = 10^{-14}$."[150] Unpacking the hieroglyphics of his equations are words that precisely state the measurable and quantifiable changes he desires to manifest in water. In Tiller's intention, the composition of water and the structure of water are two entirely different states, which he knows will lead to different understandings of how water may interact with itself and other matter. A materials science concept known as "epitaxy," the ability of an existing crystalline structure to control the structural orientation of crystal growth, is one example of how information is transmitted in other ways distinct from just chemical additions. Tiller knows that water structure can change properties vastly more easily and dramatically than by chemical reaction alone. In effect, Tiller expands the language of water beyond the language of chemistry, freely revising his information creation and rewriting it if necessary until it feels right.[151]

• Including in the final analysis, the subjective feeling he uses as a guide: peacefulness. His creative process then ends with his written declaration: "Thy will be done."

That the process ends with "Thy will be done" is, I feel, a powerful prayer. Tiller invokes The Lord's Prayer, which is among the greatest of them all. No one who reads this can fail to catch something of its majesty and timelessness. It is like the string through the beads of thought. It is an article of faith. It packs a punch. It is Tiller's "spiritual science" and, in a sense, he asks to see the Truth. He opens a line of communication with the Source of all revelatory thought. Maybe that is the same thing as consulting your conscience. Maybe that is the same thing as a discussion with God.

It is easy to overlook one aspect of this process. The most important part of the process is that the intention is written down. There is something magical about writing things down. Why is writing so effective? It allows intention, a mental process, to be made active. There is more oomph when the written word is rendered physical on paper. Writing strengthens the intention. He doesn't use word processing, emails, tweets, or even a computer. As he sees it, creating information on paper sharpens focus. It seems to me Tiller's action of writing says something about the relationship between intention—a creative aspect—and the physical act of writing.

I am sure you are just as struck as I am by Tiller's protocol. He is a man convinced of the necessity for God to be at the center of all life. He sees no difference between a marvelous scientific discovery and a prayer. Tiller combines the separate strengths of spiritual practice and science and comes up with his radically subjective protocol. Will it work?

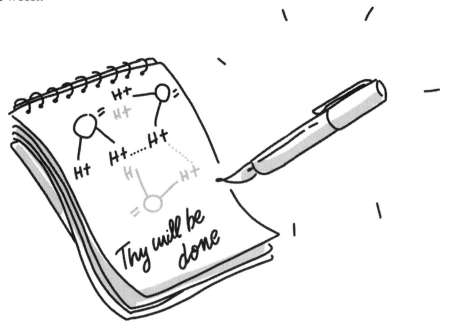

[23]
"We were assisted by the Unseen."
The Crazy Ridiculous Idea of a Device:
Do You Have the Right Stuff?

Creating an intention is one thing; prying open the secrets of how your intention manifests is an altogether different endeavor. Tiller studies the strengths and flaws of holding an intention, not for a few seconds or a few minutes, but for up to forty-five minutes, in one unbroken focus.

The mind is swift, changing in a split second, with new streams of thought, a dozen new directions. It seems beyond our conscious control. If intention can't overcome the natural tendency of your mind to wander ceaselessly—and you have to admit, it's incredibly fast—you have a problem with the protocol design. There is a second, even bigger issue. When he developed the protocol, Tiller had no idea how much time it would take for the effects of intention to manifest. Would it take days for the intention to do its job? Weeks? Months? It's impossible to hold one intention continuously or repeatedly for so long.[152]

As Tiller conceptualized his experiment, he became familiar with the enormous odds. To overcome the obstacle of holding an intention for long periods, he resolutely looked at all options. Being a superbly skilled adept at inner self-management, the answer he finally struck upon was one unlikely to have occurred to anyone but him.

The gas discharge experiments described in Pillar 1 had established that humans can alter gas ionization rates solely by their intention without physical contact. Tiller also knew the psychoenergetic research data from labs like the PEAR research group showing that humans, from a distance, could impact a machine in a given direction by their intention. With this scientific evidence, he asked himself a momentous question: Could an object, such as a simple machine, be a stable repository of subtle energy intention information? "We had to have a way to objectify human intention," he explained to me. "The way I thought about it was to hold a single thought, like an adept, but with a device. This machine must hold intention information. I felt that's worth trying. If we can successfully stably imprint a device, meaning it would hold the intention information without leaking away, it would be a game-changer."

The device Tiller used was a simple circuit housed in a small plastic box, seven inches long by three inches wide and one inch tall, with a power output of less than one-millionth of a watt. An apparatus imprinted with human intention was "activated" with subtle energy to a metastable state "excited" above equilibrium.[153] Such a metastable device, Tiller reasoned, could be used, like a laser, to send out information to the intended target, continuously, without interruption. Over time, the device would slowly run back down to equilibrium.

An imprinted device is better than humans who can change their mind, vary their depth of concentration, and even fall asleep. The trick in Tiller's design was to eliminate drifting. It was like forging a symbiotic relationship between man and machine. Furthermore, the notion of the device as a laser had something symbolic about it, something metaphysical. A laser is a light. We can all use something sent out with light to guide us along our way.[154] After all, we're all in the dark much of the time. An activated device illuminates the intention and sends it on. This idea grabbed me.

In the overall scheme, intention research—held to be the domain of the brain—was finally to be made accessible by this method. Can anyone think of a better implication? If things didn't go as planned on paper, well then, as Tiller says, "we shan't have proved anything." But the device could be well within the range of plausibility. Tiller was going for the moonshot.

Tiller moved to the next problem: the imprinting process.

The first experiments at Stanford University were conducted in his physics lab, a place brimming with meters and gauges and all manner of equipment. Tiller, however, saw the space through uncommon eyes. He saw intention turn the lab into a space that would drink in subtle energies, like a parched sponge.

Three Stanford graduate students in the postdoctoral engineering program joined Tiller to make up the first imprinting team. The members of the team weren't newbies, nor were they old hands yet. If they had any small advantage, it was that they all had reputations as both brainiacs and highly experienced meditators. On the outside, to you and me, the students would appear no different than any other university student. Their eyes, their faces, their dress gave nothing away. Our perceptions about a person's inner "beingness" and level of consciousness can be deceiving. In self-development, the students were skilled lifelong practitioners of meditation. Tiller demanded that of himself and his team. For successful imprinting, only people who know, deep down, that they had the right stuff to succeed would sign up for such a rigorous protocol.

With such a difficult yet delicate experimental protocol, who would you choose to be on your team? How do you select them? From only outer appearances or their academic resumes, one cannot separate them. But we are familiar with people who are "pumper-uppers" and those who are "drainer-downers."

For the imprinting process, Tiller and his team settled into chairs around a lab table, each like a member of an orchestra, tuning their inner instruments for the right pitch, the perfect note on the inner strings, with eyes closed, and senses exquisitely in unison. Then silence. The air clear, like you could drink it in. In the middle of the circle, a device was placed, switched on, ready for the soundless notes of intention's subtle energy.

Tiller's voice intoned. Each time there would be wonder in his voice, as though it was his first time, even though he had imprinted many times. He read the intention statement while each member channeled his or her readiness, which gave way to a relaxed and useful hyperawareness. Like music playing inside, the song of the words "Thy will be done" lingering, suspended, feeling its way into each heart.

The imprinting process made its ascent, climbing higher and higher in ever-expanding circles. There was a communion with one another, with the device, with the Unseen. Thirty minutes later, the students came out of meditation with Tiller affirming again, "Thy will be done!" to conclude the session. Each member returned feeling full, even rejuvenated. The euphoric rush of collective meditation never got old. Nothing else needed to be explained.

Later, I asked about the euphoria during the imprinting. Tiller said: "Our experimental results have a lot to do with subjective variables like emotions and meaning, which is another way to say love. It feels like the Unseen is doing the heavy lifting. We are assisted in this process."

I know what you're thinking: Wow. I mean WOW! This is something entirely new. I had never encountered anything like it. As your friend who's been there, I report expansive feelings, soaring to great heights. (Note that these are all spatial attributes.) Tiller is fun, no doubt about it. When you've been in medicine with austere research agendas and been lectured about objectivity, this new experience is both a revelation and emancipation. Witness one of the imprinting sessions, and the outside world—clinical demands, the papers to write, life at home and all its worries—falls away. It lasted, I regret to say, for a day, and then I was back in the twenty-first century, reductionist as ever.

How did they know the device was successfully activated or imprinted? I remembered my own exasperation with incomplete records, understanding for the first time the difficulty of being an eyewitness to anything unusual. Objectivity is all very well, but it is possible only when you can describe your experience in terms of standard weights and measures. We do not know the frequency and intensity of the intention, cannot provide an accurate record of its size, shape, or weight. I believe it is nevertheless meaningful to report my investigation. Tiller's protocol seems to blur the boundary between man and machine, like playing a musical instrument or driving your car. Tiller calls the imprinted device an "Intention Host Device," or IHD.[155]

Scientific logic and emotion have no contradiction. Science is thought of as objective. That is the culture. Yet science is also subjective. Feelings catalyze, complement, and reinforce each other. Tiller is not the first scientist to emphasize that he is being assisted by the Unseen. On his deathbed in 1879, James Clerk Maxwell said:

> What is done
> by what is called myself is, I feel,
> done by something greater
> than myself in me.[156]

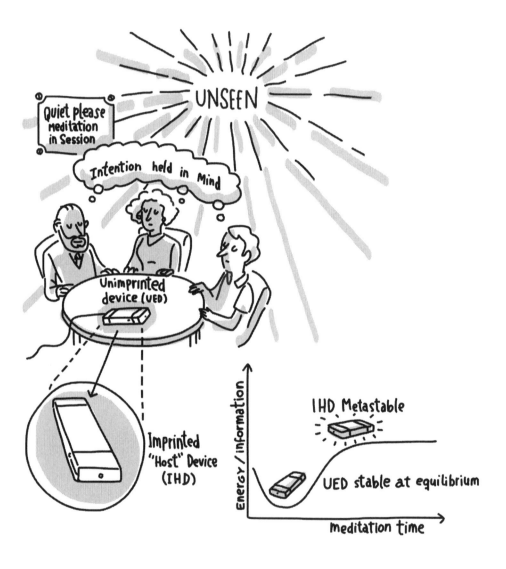

[24]
"We lost our controls."
The Problem of Good Controls in Subtle Energy Research:
The Granny Effect

Science is about testing a hypothesis to see whether it's right or wrong. A key element of good experimental design is a control, a set-up without active treatment. It is best illustrated by an example. Let's say you want to test whether a device helps to reduce arthritis pain. You have two groups of arthritis sufferers: one, the active group, will get the device that delivers pain-relieving treatment, while the other, the control group, will receive an identical "dummy" device that does not deliver the treatment. A control serves as your baseline or reference in research. At the end of the study, you get results from both groups. For the device to be considered effective and to eliminate other variables (like the placebo effect or measurement errors), you have to show that the active group found the real device reduced their pain significantly more than did the group who had the dummy device. Therefore, controls help increase the reliability of conclusions drawn from your results.

In subtle energy research, scientists recognize the challenges and extra precautions necessary in the design set up between active and control groups, especially when people are involved. For example, when investigating an energy healer, to circumvent any placebo effect, labs use animals or cell cultures since they don't seem to have opinions one way or another about healing or healers.[157] Moreover, researchers reason that using animals (rodents) and cells not only eliminates psychosocial factors of expectations and beliefs, but "extraneous healing intention" is also minimized. For example, we can be pretty sure that nobody's grandmother—let alone her church group, is praying for cells in an experiment, as the case might be with hospitalized human subjects.[158]

What this means is that scientists understand that subtle energies appear "intelligent" (how else does Granny's prayer identify you in among your group of friends?), that these intentions traverse great distances (Granny lives on the other side of the country), and these intentions are magnified by the collective power of people working together (her church group, whose "dose" of the intention seems to be magnitudes greater) and somehow go through the walls of your home to reach you. After all, she did not call you on the phone, and her intention is not transmitted through a phone line by electromagnetic waves. These are worthy strategies, but they still miss fundamental issues that Tiller uncovered. He found that you cannot shield or block the subtle energy; it exists within a different set of rules.

Given this background, let's turn to Tiller's research on intention. To compare the effects of intention, a control unimprinted electronic device (UED) is necessary. Identical experiments are set up. In one, the IHD (factor being tested) is applied to a target (such as water) and in another, the UED serves as the control. This seems straightforward. After all, when we see two devices, the IHD and UED, separated without physical contact, we'd expect the UED to be a suitable control.[159] But something else happened.

During the water studies, Tiller found that the UED also changed the pH of its own water sample, suggesting that the intention charge is somehow transferred from the IHD to the UED. This happened within a few days to a week, thereby ruining the control for the target experiments. It appears that, even for the devices in the "off" condition, a transfer of information occurs! How does the transfer happen? We don't know. Tiller was flummoxed. Initial frustration gave way to a hunch that they were encountering a kind of connectivity between the active and control devices which Tiller called "macroscopic information entanglement." This information entanglement, which I term the "Granny effect," cannot be blocked. Nature is far more complex than the variables we think we have controlled for.

How could they adjust? Over research meetings, he and the lab crew worked out details of the overall design to reduce "cross-talk" between the devices. He tapped his longtime buddy Walter Dibble, an experimentalist extraordinaire. Dibble had been with Tiller labs since his doctoral program. First off, carefully isolating the unimprinted (UED) and imprinted devices (IHD) from each other was essential for reducing transfer of the intention-charge between them.

Next Dibble experimented with various types of shielding methods.[160] Ambient electromagnetic fields could be spreading the IHD signal, acting as augmented carrier-waves and transferring information to the unimprinted device. After all, electromagnetism—that is, ambient EMF—surrounds everything and likely interacts with subtle energy information.

Ordinary kitchen aluminum foil proved an effective block for photons (the particle aspect of light). Next, the real trick: Faraday cages constructed from fine copper wire mesh (a 0.16-inch grid) in a cylindrical geometry measuring twelve inches in diameter blocked electromagnetic radiation (the wave aspect of light), such as radio waves and microwaves. The IHD and UED were stored in these electrically grounded Faraday cages. Using these procedures, the team observed via pH that they were able to maintain a viable intention imprint on the IHD and no detectable imprint on the UED for about three months, enough time for experiments to proceed with suitable controls.[161] They now had a way to use the UED.

The aluminum foil-wrapped devices were separately shipped on different days via Federal Express to their laboratory destination two thousand miles away in Minnesota. On arrival at the experimental lab, they were immediately placed in separate, electrically grounded Faraday cages until used in the experiments. The personnel at the receiving lab were "blind" not only to the imprint directive but also to whether they had an IHD or UED. This blinding served as a further control.

The "cross-talk" between an imprinted device and controls pointed to a broader truth that awaited discovery. Tiller reflected: "As I thought more about it, because the Faraday cages are electrically grounded, there is no electromagnetism. It means that there is another channel for communication in nature."

What seemed to have been a nuisance in their protocol—the IHD and UED cross-talk—forced them to troubleshoot the information entanglement effects and ultimately turned out to be crucial for Tiller's future work.

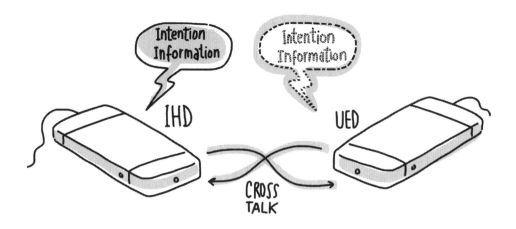

[25]
"We can affect materials like water with purely our intention."
The Frugal Science of Human Intention

Tiller and fellow scientist Walter Dibble set up the first target experiments aiming to test whether a device (IHD) imprinted with an intention could bring about a change in water's pH in the intended direction.[162] Water pH is subject to several factors that must be carefully controlled for. Published thermodynamic data of water pH from other labs served as the reference point. The equilibrium pH at a given water temperature could be readily calculated from established thermodynamic data taking into account carbon dioxide dissolved in water.

Another element was evaporation (an unavoidable factor in order to maintain equilibrium with air in long-term studies), which could change the composition of water and introduce spurious effects. They used purified water that exceeded the American Society of Testing and Materials standards for ultrapure water, thereby ensuring the composition and that consequently the pH of water did not change during extended periods. The pH of purified water in equilibrium with air at 25 °C is around 5.66.

The experimental equipment permitted a high signal-to-noise discrimination with protection against technical malfunctions. Tiller employed Accumet 150 pH meters and fast-response, high-performance glass combination electrodes to monitor both water temperature and pH with measurement accuracy of 0.001 pH units. They performed extensive and regular calibrations with buffer standards (pH 7, pH 10, and pH 4) to confirm the stability of the system and its conformity to theoretical expectations.

Tiller's engineering and materials science expertise gave him an advantage where it was needed. Tiller also monitored the air temperature of the laboratory with thermometers inside the Faraday cage and outside the experimental setup at different locations around the room. Data points like air temperature are not routinely recorded in intention research. To him, not only was the target important but, monitoring the laboratory space was crucial, too. The pieces began to fall into place.

From the very first day, as the IHD was unwrapped and placed a precise six inches from the purified water inside a Faraday cage, computer monitoring of the digital data outputs commenced immediately at one-minute intervals, with data sets collected daily. In a separate room down the hallway, an identical setup for the UED control was underway. A third setup without any device (with only the water and pH electrodes in a Faraday cage) isolated in a different room from the IHD and UED also served as a control.

The goal of the first of the target experiments was to increase (or decrease) the pH of water one full unit by pure intention, without chemical additions. A pH change of one unit may not seem like a big deal; however, consider that the pH range value is just 0 to 14 units. Orange juice has a pH of 5; Clorox bleach is basic or alkaline with a pH of 12. The pH of human blood is extraordinarily steady at 7.40, just on the alkaline side of neutrality (pH 7). In real terms, a magnitude of change of one unit for water was chosen purposely, being well out of the range of "random noise" effects.

Intention research has a way of feeling both gradual and surprisingly sudden. The initial blips on water pH measurements bobbed up and down as expected, as it equilibrated with the carbon dioxide in the air during the first twenty to forty minutes. Then the thin line of the pH settled down at equilibrium and the waiting began.

In the set up with the IHD imprinted with a directive to increase pH, the water's pH started its slow ascent, as though an unseen hand cranked it along. Within two months, the water had answered: the hydrogen ions, which make water acidic, decreased by a factor of log ten (1 pH unit) from baseline with no other intervention.

Similar results occurred for the IHD with the directive to lower the water's pH by one unit: the pH *decreased*. On the other hand, the water pH results for the UED in a Faraday cage were almost identical to those of the no device control. After the first forty minutes, once the water pH settled to equilibrium pH of around 5.70, the two controls stayed constant.

Can we hit pause for a second and acknowledge how bonkers this is? It's full-on bananas, a rewrite of the history books. I believe the word is *yowza*.

Most would argue that it is not possible for a human's intention to produce physically detectable differences in a common laboratory measurement. But the experiment went further. To capture such a remarkable effect with a physical device (IHD), which itself would be considered impossible, means the probability would be the product of two highly improbable events. As Tiller and Dibble wrote in their paper "Electronic Device-Mediated pH Changes in Water" in the *Journal of Scientific Exploration:* "We challenge this conventional wisdom [of improbability] and choose to let the experimental data speak for itself."[163] A difference in water pH of such magnitude as one unit between prediction and observation had the potential to reshape what we know, or think we know, about nature and ourselves.[164] Tiller and Dibble were "blown away."

The water pH could have changed due to any number of reasons. Maybe the ionic bonds between the H_2O molecules were getting weaker somehow and sharing electrons more readily, or perhaps water molecules were colliding and sliding in distinct ways, exchanging electrons and producing fewer or more hydronium ions according to the primary intention. Chemists will tell you it takes some energy—that is, ΔG (Gibbs free energy)—for the ion exchange necessary to move water to a higher or lower pH. When water has an injection of ΔG, the molecules speed up, and more molecules are bumping into each other and exchanging ions. The probability of pH change is raised. But there was no traditional energy or chemical input into the experimental system.

To explain this, Tiller had an initial hunch. But even he was gobsmacked as to the answer that emerged. He knew nothing of what was yet to be revealed by his full data set. Mother Nature had more cards to play than he could know.

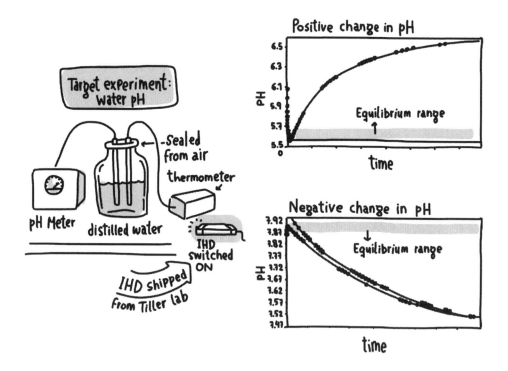

[26]
"Intention can enhance biological enzyme function."
The Case of Alkaline Phosphatase Chemical Potential

If "change water, change your world" has whetted your appetite, then you may be asking what the functional relevance of these water pH changes is. It was a tall order to change water in any parameter exclusively by intention, but now that it had been achieved, the question naturally arose as to whether biological materials might be similarly amenable as targets. After all, the major component of functioning biological systems is water, which is the medium of aqueous solutions such as blood and digestive juices.

Tiller teamed up with a Stanford University colleague Michael Kohane. By formal training, Kohane is a biochemist and geneticist. He is an expert in enzyme functions. When Kohane learned of Tiller's proposal to use an IHD to enhance enzyme function, he was not sure such a "crazy" protocol could work. But he had the know-how and expertise in biology that Tiller needed. They were a match made in science heaven.

They chose alkaline phosphatase (ALP) as their target. As the name implies, ALP works best in an alkaline environment. It is ubiquitous in your body, present in nearly all tissues and at particularly high levels in the liver and bones. The ALP level is routinely reported as part of the "chem-panel," a blood test done millions of times every day as one of the most frequent doctors' orders. ALP reflects liver and bone health.

Enzymes are the workhorses of the body and make biochemical reactions go faster. Put another way, enzymes speed up reaction rates.[165] Chemical reactions require some energy input to get going. It's like a log of wood needs some ΔG, in the form of a match, to ignite it. Enzymes "light up" chemical reactions in your cells by reducing the required level of activation energy. ALP's job is to link up with its target molecule and "decouple" or separate a phosphate from the target molecule. The end product of the reaction is a new molecule plus an individual phosphate group. ALP is not consumed in the reaction and is ready to get working on more substrate.

What do we mean by reaction rate? The rate means how fast enzyme ALP can change the target to the two end products. The human body has a variety of natural triggers for increasing the thermodynamic activity of ALP. For example, if the liver is obstructed by a gallstone, its response is to make more ALP. The rate is also dependent on factors like the concentration of starting molecules and the local cellular environment where the reaction takes place.

The central hypothesis Tiller and Kohane set about to test is whether the speed of the ALP reaction, its thermodynamic activity, can be affected by intention alone under controlled conditions.

Enzyme kinetics have been extensively studied, and Tiller and Kohane used well-validated methods for the intention experiment. The thermodynamic activity of ALP was determined via reflective spectroscopy utilizing the target 4-nitrophenyl phosphate (4-NPP). This is colorless, but 4-nitrophenol (4-NP), the product after ALP action, is yellow.[166] Thus, ALP reactivity can be followed continuously by observing the rate of increase of yellow color spectrophotometrically.

Suppose we want to measure enzyme activity as did Tiller. We use a fixed amount of ALP—say, five copies in our glass vessel. Each copy of ALP can catalyze (churn out product) at a rate of ten reactions per second. The maximum rate is fifty reactions per second; that is, we cannot increase the rate above fifty by giving more starting molecules. We also assume that all our solutions are behaving ideally, and that ALP is stable and not degraded. Furthermore, we make sure that environmental factors are constant, that no external factors are messing things up, and that all reactions in our lab are thermodynamically stable.

As with the water pH experiment, we set up three experiments: first, an IHD to increase ALP activity; second, a control with the UED; and third, as a further control, a set up with no device present. Experiments with devices are in Faraday cages to screen out ambient EMF, and the no-device set up is on the tabletop without a Faraday cage. The ALP in each vessel is exposed to the devices—IHD, UED, or none—for thirty minutes while color changes are monitored spectrophotometrically.

The set up with no device takes a longer time to yield yellow product than the IHD. Good. With the UED, the time to the product is even longer than no device. We are puzzled.

With the IHD, there is an increase of more than 15 percent of the thermodynamic activity of ALP! It's like saying the five copies of enzyme were doing the work of six, and product is churned out at a speedier rate. We repeat the experiment with the IHD again the following day and find the thermodynamic activity of ALP is even greater.

The first question is why the UED control is worse than no device being present. Tiller felt that the EMF produced by the UED likely affects ALP activity more than environmental EMF. The UED's electromagnetic field appears to add to the "stress" for biological material.[167]

Additionally, part of the results strikes an odd note to Tiller's engineer ear, if only for its inexplicability. Usually when measuring enzyme activity in a lab, it does not matter whether we make the measurement on day one or day two. After all, when you have your blood tested, it doesn't affect your results whether it's a Monday or a Tuesday. With the IHD, the ALP activity is greater on day two versus day one.[168] All things being equal, there should be no difference at all. The IHD does indeed change something about the environment, but how? And why are the results better on day two? This is a mystery waiting to be solved.

What does an increase in ALP mean in practical terms? I don't know what it would mean for a living animal or human, but I am willing to wager that ALP releasing phosphate faster could lead to better energy production. Among all the target molecules ALP acts on, the most ubiquitous among living systems is adenosine triphosphate (ATP). ALP removes phosphate to release energy.

Together with the water pH experiments, the enzyme target experiment accelerated Tiller's research of intention effects. He was just beginning. Intention can do impressive things.

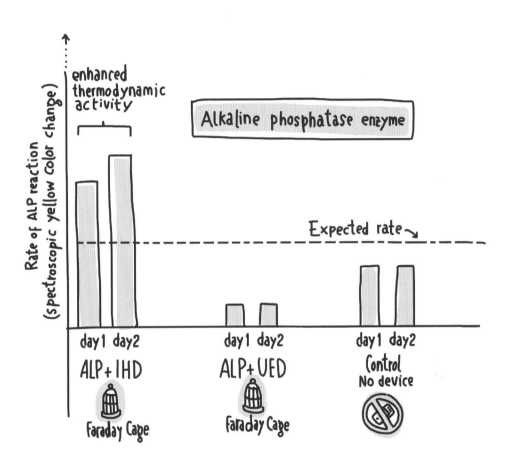

[27]
"The happy fruit flies."
Human Intention and a Living System

Tiller decided to put his protocol to the supreme test: determining whether intention could benefit a living system, under lab conditions, and with controls. This test had magnitudes greater significance for he was dealing with a form of life.

Teaming up again with Michael Kohane, they chose a biological superstar, the fruit fly (*Drosophila melanogaster, "Drosophila"* hereafter). Drosophila has a characteristic like no other species: its life cycle from fly to egg to larva to adult occurs in a span of an ultra-short fourteen days, and eggs hatch in just a day. It's almost as if they were *designed* to help scientists.[169] Put a male and female *Drosophila* together, and a fortnight later new offspring hatch and a new generation takes wing. Fruit fly reproduction is exceptionally reliable, with two parents producing predictable offspring, meaning guaranteed eggs and larvae.

The central hypothesis is that intention can affect the life cycle of the *Drosophila*. Tiller's intention reads: "To increase the ATP energy ratio to inactive energy such that the larval developmental time to adult is twenty-five percent shorter or better."

With the right environment, fruit flies were eager to reveal their secrets. The lab was at the perfect temperature, a steady 18° to 25°C, and the fruit fly's favorite foods, such as yeast and sugar, were in plentiful supply. As though being called to "be fruitful" and multiply, they coupled in the tiny tubes, two-by-two, and reveling in domestic bliss, started new families.[170] The pregnant female, her long-pointed abdomen bulging with precious eggs, laid thirty to fifty per day throughout her two-week lifetime. Within twenty-four to thirty hours, the eggs hatched into larvae. In six or seven days, the larvae increased around a thousand-fold in weight to their adult size. Development time is an indicator of fitness, since healthier offspring take less time to mature into adults.

Thirty newly hatched larvae, plump and glossy, looking like tiny white worms, were taken by Kohane and placed in a single vial with food. Fifteen vials were carefully prepared this way. The vials were randomly set up near one of four experimental setups, all in the same room: 1) on a table in the lab environment (control); 2) inside a Faraday cage with an IHD; 3) inside a Faraday cage with a UED (control); and 4) in a Faraday cage without a device control. Careful daily inspections and daily counts were done as adults began appearing.

The results: larvae inside the Faraday cage without any device had the best, most rapid developmental time compared with the other three setups. The IHD and environmental tied in second place, followed by the UED in last (worst) place. The larva in the presence of the IHD developed faster than did the UED control. Why did the flies with IHD have slower developmental times than the Faraday-caged no-device setup? Tiller's hunch was that electromagnetic fields—ambient or from devices—were detrimental to the health and fitness of *Drosophila*.[171] The Faraday cage is good housing, as it screens out ambient electromagnetic fields (EMF). The IHD's intention compensates, to some extent, for the EMF generated by the electronics housed in it. It has better outcomes than the unimprinted device (UED), which had the worst developmental times.

What is the pathway for *Drosophila's* enhanced ATP production? Could mitochondria, the "ATP manufacturing plant" of the cell, chug out more ATP? The experimental work extended into the possible mechanisms. It is shown that a key molecule in metabolism and flow of energy in biological systems is positively enhanced in the fruit fly exposed to the IHD.[172] The *Drosophila* has a natural maturation rhythm already built into the memory of the insect's cells. I am therefore particularly impressed that this rhythm can be tuned by the IHD in Tiller's labs in order to produce a new series of perfectly timed developmental patterns. It seems that the fly responds to even the subtlest scraps of information.

What could a fruit fly have in common with humans? *Drosophila* shares an astounding 60 percent of human DNA. Up to 75 percent of human disease genes have a recognizable match in fruit flies, including Alzheimer's, diabetes, various cancers, and even autism. Fruit flies offer a cheap, fast pipeline to understanding complex biological questions that can be translated to medical applications. Tiller had success in helping *Drosophila*. Can intention help one of many vexing medical problems that plague humans? Can intention research be bridged, or translated, from the lab to real-world medicine? In Tiller's mind, the target experimental data reveal what his work could accomplish.

One aspect is striking to me. In his science as in his meditations, Tiller follows the path of the heart. He did not fail on that account with the fruit fly. It brought to my mind that essential of scriptural teachings, Matthew 7:16 playfully modified: "Ye shall know them by their 'fruit flies.'"

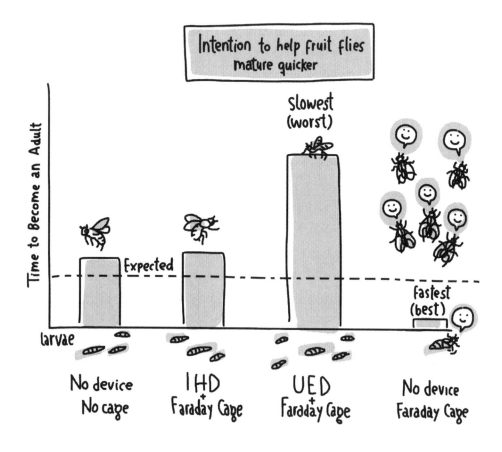

[28]
"Objects can have 'intelligence.'"
Target Experiments Turn Science Upside Down

I know from experience that readers of this book will be disproportionately interested in the device. I might be declared a dimwit, a consumer of Tiller Kool-Aid, or worse. The argument can be boiled down to its pivotal question: Is an IHD experiment legitimate science, as opposed to a pipe dream? I want to be perfectly clear: I don't believe in fantasy. To help you weigh whether the device is sound science against the possibility that the IHD is some hocus pocus, here are my answers to frequently asked questions:

FAQ #1: Why use a device in the first place?

An obstacle is a very good teacher. Encountering seemingly insurmountable barriers to holding an intention continuously, Tiller feels it is beneficial to have some aids, like an IHD which is "on" 24/7 with a steady pulse, like a laser, of subtle energy information. Tiller calls his version a "Model-T," humorously likening it to the first affordable car manufactured by the Henry Ford company. Training wheels do their job and take you from point A to point B in the target experiment until the metastable device runs down to equilibrium and, just like a car, needs to be refueled and topped up with re-imprinting, ready for another round. In future, such devices may be like Ferraris! This is not as crazy as it sounds.

FAQ #2: Is there something special about Tiller's choice of the plastic box?

Any object can be imprinted. In this sense, his device is no more special than the shirt you're wearing.[173] For purposes of a scientific protocol, Tiller used a type of device nearly identical to any little commercial electronic device, like a TV remote control. He special-ordered it from a manufacturer so that it could be readily available for other scientists in other labs to reproduce his experimental results. This type of device allows for a standardized experimental protocol.

FAQ #3: Why does Tiller say the IHD is "intelligent"?

The experimental data speaks for itself. I cannot think of a better word than "intelligence." Some of you will protest. However, it's compelling that not only does an IHD act as a repository of human intention but it will only have the result of its imprinted directive and not something else. With each experiment replicated hundreds of times, the human instruction came into manifestation via the IHD. The UEDs do not demonstrate that capability. A device *requires* human subtle energy and human *intelligence* (or information) to be activated.[174]

FAQ #4: Are there other real-world examples of intelligent machines?

We have all experienced those strange moments when things seem to take on a life of their own. Valued possessions return to their owners, lost items reappear in unlikely places, and computers misbehave.[175] Are we investing objects with a life force through the attention we give them? It seems that matter can absorb emotional "fingerprints." This gains some credence from the informal testimony of laboratory operators, who frequently speak of achieving a state of "resonance" with the device during successful operation. It is no different than driving a car or playing a musical instrument. The boundary between animate and inanimate becomes blurred. Even our user-friendly electronic "personal" assistants are given names such as Siri, Alexa, and Cortana.

FAQ #5: Is the IHD good for anything else?

Good question. You're thinking like an engineer and bridge builder.

FAQ #6: What studies have been done on the device?

Tiller understands that the device isn't the thing to scrutinize; it's the results, like the eddy in the stream of clear intention. It is not a random process, with skill and intent increasing the odds of successful imprinting. Tiller also reminds us to shift interest from details to the big picture and to focus on the overall qualities of what the target experimental data signify. We don't need to know every detail of why an IHD works to take advantage of it.

FAQ #7: Is there some sort of magic with the device?

Whether we see something as magic is about perspective. In the movie *The Gods Must Be Crazy,* an African Bushman considers an empty Coca-Cola bottle to be magical.[176] Even if he were shown that it is a useful object because it can carry water, he might still revere or pray to the bottle or feel heartbroken if the bottle cracks. In his worldview, the bottle is unique and unexpected, and therefore magical. Likewise, an IHD may appear to have magical qualities, attracting more scrutiny and admiration than necessary.

FAQ #8: What is the difference between the IHD and artificial intelligence?

In my experience when talking about the target experiments, people easily fall into a comparison between artificial intelligence, or AI, and Tiller's IHD. The keyword in AI is "artificial"; it is a machine programmed by algorithms. There is no imminent technological magic bullet that is truly revolutionary. Bill Buxton, a father of the touch screen and a principal researcher at Microsoft, says: "The people who have the tech skills may not have the cultural and social skills. It's only when you get all those skills together that you get the perfect storm for the next breakthrough."[177] I would add to Buxton's caution: in people with the tech skills, a high level of consciousness is needed for truly innovative AI technology.

I feel there is something more pressing that is unspoken about AI. AI can make us passive and dependent, as basic human actions are turned over to machines. The best of us are prone to slackness. This is true for our conscious endeavors and also subconscious work. We can slip deeper into unconsciousnesss, and the information we create becomes lackluster. It is a mark of laziness that in AI's growth we lose consciousness of its existence and only awaken to it when we discover its disastrous effects. Consider the prospect of human species becoming *Homo piger,* the lazy man.

With an IHD, humans are supercharged, in control, and alert. They are pumped up. The IHD is magnificent in its real implications for the larger Truth of who we can become. *It* is the game changer.

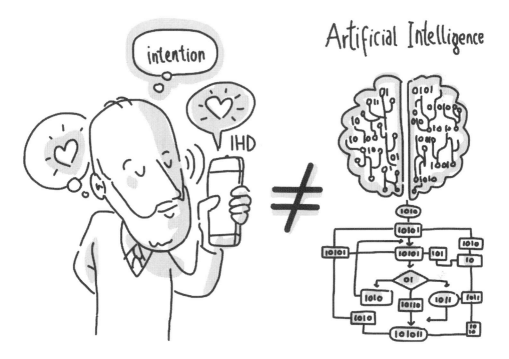

It so happens that the work which is likely to be our most durable monument, and to convey some knowledge of us to the most remote posterity, is a work of bare utility; not a shrine, not a fortress, not a palace, but a bridge.

—Montgomery Schuyler

in *Harper's Weekly,* May 24, 1883[178]

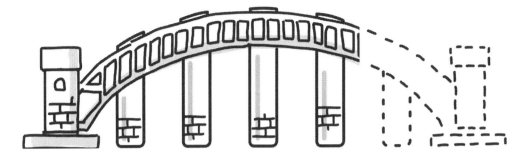

BRIDGE PILLAR 5:
Of Physical Space and Dual Realities:
Beyond the Speed of Light

SPACE remains the highest Divinity that is in any sense know-
able, however dim that knowledge may be.

–FRANKLIN MERRELL-WOLFF,
***Pathways through to Space. An Experiential Journal**[179]*

When men doubt, it is often because they are troubled by destiny,
what is firm to touch or appears hard to the eye. The infinities of
smallness they know nothing about, such as the solidity of gases or
the vast spaces between the universes which make a lump of sugar.
They trust their limited perceptions of the world about them
and are entirely ignorant of the rapidly changing conceptions of
matter. Men need to look more, not less, to science and such men
as Eddington, who are not confounded by the visible universe.

–ANONYMOUS,
from *Letters of the Scattered Brotherhood* by Mary Strong[180]

We appear to be entering a period of human evolution in which certain qualities of the human being appear to be able to change, or deform, basic quantities [of space and time]. Thus, our set of laws or consistency relationships will have to change to embrace this new experience. It isn't as if the old laws are wrong and need to be thrown out—no more than Newton was wrong when Einstein came along and showed that the laws of gravitation had to be altered when one adopted a frame of reference for observation that moved at velocities approaching the velocity of light.

—WILLIAM A. TILLER[181]

[29]
"Physical space is malleable to human intention."
The Next Big Thing in Space Is Closer Than You Think:
Good Vibrations

Tiller was now in possession of something priceless. His lab had coordinated data sets from multiple replications of the water pH experiments. His results, let's face it, look mysterious and anomalous. A piece of the puzzle of the riddle of the large intention effects lay in plain sight, an unexpected surprise. His impeccable lab setup rewarded Tiller with data that scientists can only dream of.

The temperature of water is a key thermodynamic variable in calculating its predicted pH under normal conditions. Specifically, water's temperature and its pH are strongly correlated. Tiller's data, on the other hand, revealed a different and strikingly unusual pattern. There was an *inverse* correlation between water pH and its temperature. Instead, strangely, the water pH correlated with the temperature of the *room* air.

Charting the data sets for these properties—water pH, water temperature, and air temperature—revealed plots showing precise waveforms. For example, the room air temperature oscillated up and down, a swing of 3 °C, a rhythm so large that the high-resolution digital thermometers' sensitivity of 0.001 °C clearly showed the unusual swings. These were not "blips" or random noise. We can stick a thermometer in a room. The air molecules tumbling around give rise to air currents, and our thermometer would record variations resembling a skein of tracings adrift without a sawtooth pattern, just like was seen in lab spaces without a device or with a UED.[182]

Could the oscillations in air temperature be originating from the IHD inside the Faraday cage? Tiller removed the IHD and water vessel. The air temperature continued to oscillate merrily away. Location of heating or air conditioning similarly didn't account for the observations. These findings served as a reminder that what Tiller and his team were investigating isn't bound to some visible spectra. It's like a ghost in the physical world. Tiller calls them "phantom" waves. He was positively confounded.

What causes waves? In physics, a wave is a disturbance in a medium that moves energy from a source. When a violin string is plucked, the air disturbance travels as sound waves to your ear. Or when you throw a pebble into a still pond, circular ripples transfer the energy outward from the spot of the pebble's impact. But the oscillations in Tiller's data set were different. They continued, as if of their own accord, without dissipating.

Tiller graphed the air temperature to orient in time and space. Typically, air temperature fluctuates with day and night cycles, called "diurnal variations." The temperature oscillations, however, continued without nighttime dips. In fact, as days and nights rolled by, the oscillations became persistent over forty thousand hours of data. This means that for more than four and a half years, the Tiller laboratories in Payson, Arizona, recorded these continuous anomalous fluctuations, demonstrating some yet unknown and undescribed property of their labs.[183]

Air temperature waveforms would be expected to dissipate and disappear unless some heat or energy is used to top them up and keep the currents going. Yet there was no heat source to drive these waves. Furthermore, waves are usually predictably localized in space, in one spot of the lab. Not these. Data from thermistors inside the Faraday cage at the pH experimental setup, at various locations around the room outside of the Faraday cage, and even outside the closed door ten feet into the hallway showed the distinctive oscillations.

Likewise, the water pH and water temperature data showed a rhythmic cadence. As the pH stepped up by 0.1 unit, the water temperature stepped down by 0.05 °C, as if in an unusual dance, moving back and forth regularly. The two properties' oscillation amplitudes were 25 times larger than the instrument measurement accuracy, so they were obvious and could be observed in some detail.

To unravel the pattern of the waveforms, Fourier transform is a key tool in an engineer's bag. Fourier analysis decomposes a wave signal into the frequencies that make it up, similar to how a musical chord can be expressed as the frequencies or pitches of its constituent notes, like harmonics.[184]

The first surprise awaited: analysis of the air temperature data from the different spatial locations around the room revealed harmonics that "nested," one into another, perfectly. The recorded frequencies of the various temperature waves were all multiples of each other on paper. Even more remarkable, Fourier analysis of the oscillations of water pH and water temperature also revealed nesting harmonics, even though the wave shapes of the two different properties were dissimilar.

After crunching the numbers in different ways to make sure that the anomalous behavior wasn't a figment of computation, a mismodeling of the data, or random noise, Tiller concluded that the observations were indeed weird (anomalous) and new in nature.

What could this mean?

At the time of his discovery, Tiller said: "It tells us that something is coherently pumping the entire laboratory space and all the instruments therein! As if one common oscillating force of unlimited extent is driving all these data probes. They are metastable. They do decay slowly but over periods of weeks to months rather than in seconds or minutes, like they would if they had something to do with [the] air."

It was as if the whole room pulsated to a beat. Surely, if we could hear the lab sing, it would be like a three-instrument orchestra of viola, violin, and cello that would have lifted us off our feet. On paper, here was a new compelling harmonic arrangement for those with eyes to see it.

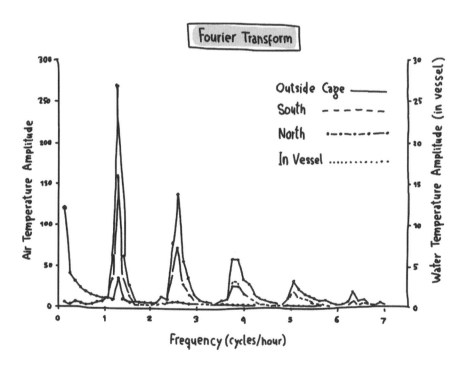

It was a broad hint that something beautiful awaited discovery. Clearly, the oscillations were some type of signal and potentially even the mechanism behind the target experimental success. They were tied together in some way. In their paper "New Experimental Data Revealing an Unexpected Dimension to Materials Science and Engineering,"[185] Tiller and Dibble discussed tantalizing new questions: Were the oscillations a necessary condition for intention effects to materialize? Where did they originate from?

They were not done yet. They wanted to be sure that the air temperature oscillations were not some artifact introduced by air currents. In nature, air temperature oscillations in space are most often caused by a layer of warm air circulating upward as cooler air flows downward, setting up a circular cell known as "Bénard convection."[186] As the air cells flow past a thermostat, they make it wobble and oscillate precisely. Therefore, either Bénard convections could be a factor or else space wasn't behaving like we think it does. The first of these possibilities is interesting. The second is like the fabled El Dorado, a physicist's city of gold come true.

There was an easy way to find out: turn on fans in the lab space to disturb the air. Such forced disturbance would dominate and homogenize the air, instantly obliterating any Bénard convections. Fans pointing at the thermostats were switched on. Astoundingly, the air temperature oscillations continued, undisturbed. This singular finding is unexplainable in conventional physics.

Tiller had found El Dorado!

The temperature waveforms were not due to air at all. They did not dissipate over thousands of hours of data recording. This pointed to one thing: The oscillations were in a nondispersive medium. In Tiller's deduction, *nondispersive* means the physical vacuum or empty space.

Tiller's great inspiration, reached after hours of replication and calculations, is this: Humans intention can affect empty space, not just the "rigid" or "flat" space, and not the "curved" relativistic space described by Einstein. His observations are remarkable and deep. They tell us that there is something special about space; not in a superficial sense, but in terms of the underlying dynamics and malleability of the very structure of nature itself and how we interact with it. Tiller described the new lab space as "conditioned." It is a reminder that space isn't an object in the same way we think of a rock or a handful of earth. The intention experiments revealed a deeper process, a wholesale redistribution of different realities. To advance the empty space properties in a conditioned lab, Tiller turned to the 1930s, an era when an eccentric and brilliant young English physicist postulated the existence of the physical vacuum.

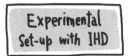

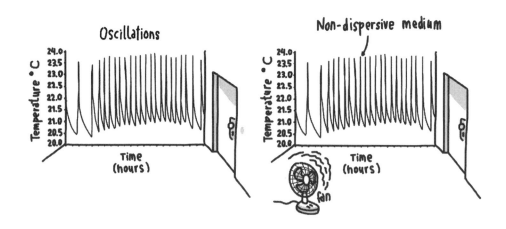

[30]
"Paul Dirac coined the term 'empty space.'"
Dirac and a Sea of Negative Energy

The 1920s and 1930s were a heady time for physics. One British scientist stood among the giants. You wouldn't have known it if you met Paul Adrian Maurice Dirac.[187] Shy, eccentric, a man of few words, Dirac's formal training was in engineering. This would prove to be an advantage: an engineer's mindset is to connect concepts, be it for better buildings, bridges, or physics theories.

Two towering theories looked incompatible: Einstein's theory of special relativity, which describes the behavior of objects moving near the speed of light, and quantum mechanics, which describes the behavior of tiny objects like electrons. An exceptional theoretician, Dirac undertook his quest to unite, like an engineer, two hugely successful theories, upgrading tried and tested designs to ones that performed better, at tighter specifications. Dirac's "playing with equations" led to formulating a relativistic quantum model of the electron. The Dirac equation was dramatic. It told physicists how to turn classical mechanical systems into quantum ones.[188] The mathematics was beautiful, linking two deep but previously unconnected theories.

From the beginning, Dirac was aware that his spectacular achievement also suffered grave problems: it had an extra set of solutions that made no physical sense since it corresponded to *negative values of energy.* In other words, the Dirac equation can be solved using *two* equally viable answers. It's like asking, what's the square root of four? If you said two, you're half right; the full answer is plus two or minus two. Every number has two square roots, one positive and one negative, and a similar doubling can occur in physics equations.

At first, Dirac didn't quite know what to do with the "negative solutions." He envisioned that the negative solutions for an electron exist in a sea of negative energy, also known as the "Dirac sea" or "physical vacuum," due to the lack of charge-based "stuff." When a cosmic ray with enough energy interacts with the vacuum, an electron is ejected so that it becomes physically observable. To conserve mass and charge, a "hole" is left behind.[189] But what characteristics do the holes have? They mark the absence of an electron, or a negative-energy electron.

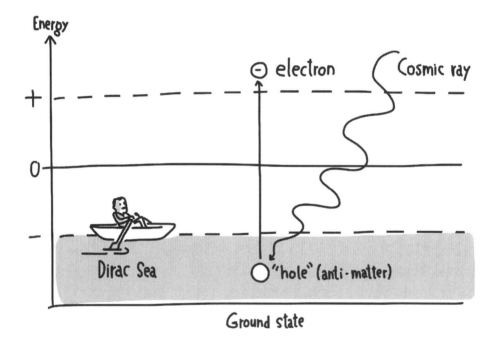

Ground state

Within the general scheme of the "negative electron sea," the absence of negative energy amounts to the presence of positive energy (two negatives make a positive). To use a familiar analogy, when debt decreases by $5, wealth increases by the same amount. Most dramatically, the Dirac equation predicted the existence of antimatter, the *mirror image* of all known particles. Every particle has a corresponding antiparticle, a doppelgänger, with the same mass but opposite charge. Dirac had theorized one of the most fascinating symmetry groups in nature, just a few years before it was successfully observed in a lab.

In 1932, Carl Anderson, a young professor at the California Institute of Technology, was studying showers of cosmic particles in a cloud chamber and saw a track left by "something positively charged, and with the same mass as an electron." In other words, he saw an "antielectron," which he went on to name the "positron" for its positive charge.[190] Anderson's observations proved the existence of the antiparticles predicted by Dirac. The very existence of antimatter hints at deep symmetries in particle physics.

Most people usually think of a vacuum as a space with nothing in it. This may seem esoteric. But physics tells you even the chair you're sitting on is mostly empty space! There is no material or physical stuff in the vacuum, so it is a *nondispersive* medium. Physics also defines the vacuum as the state in which all fields have their lowest possible energy or ground state.[191] Once a field or energy perturbs the vacuum, particles like electrons, the Higgs boson, and others come into being. The fields are always there, even when they're not excited to a higher-energy state to create a particle. A vacuum without any particles still has fields, but they are simply not excited.

It's worth noting the nexus between physics and metaphysics in Dirac's theory of matter arising from empty space. In 1939, physicist, mathematician, and mystic Franklin Merrell-Wolff wrote: "Matter and form constitute a state of relative vacuity or nothingness in the essential sense. It is interesting to note that we are now not far from a position formulated by the young English physicist Dirac, though he reached this view by means of a quite different approach."[192] Dirac arrived at the relationship between matter and empty space by equations. Merrell-Wolff, on the other hand, reached a similar position by meditation. In his meditations, he understood that the physical sciences and his self-development are "not far" from each other. One lab is outer, while the other lab is inner. They can both arrive at the Truth about our Universe.

Dirac is also remembered for his brilliant work on the electron charge and magnetic fields. Take an ordinary fridge magnet. It has a north pole and a south pole. In other words, it is dipolar. If you cut your magnet in half, you'll have two magnets, each with a north pole and south pole. You cut your two magnets in half again and you have four dipolar magnets. You can continue the process, cutting the magnet into smaller and smaller pieces, until you reach the electron with its electric charge. Electric charge spinning on its axis generates a tiny magnet. Orbiting electrons are dipolar magnets. The Dirac equation described the electron spin or magnetic moment and his theory furnished a new connection between electricity and the weakest possible magnetic charge. Atoms can act as magnets and, consequently, they can be considered analogous to a tiny compass needle.

The magnet also has a force field, represented by field lines (flowing from the positive north pole to the negative south pole in concentric arcs). In a magnetic field, denoted by symbol H, a north pole and south pole "look" the same. In contrast, we are familiar with an *electric* monopole, although we know it by its more common name: electric charge. Electric monopoles exist in the form of particles that have a positive or negative charge, such as protons or electrons. Opposite electric charges attract and like charges repel via the interaction of electric fields which are defined as running from positive to negative. These positive and negative designations are arbitrary labels for the two opposite electric charges.

On examination, magnetism appears analogous to electricity, as noted already, there exists a magnetic field with a direction defined as running from north to south. The parallel breaks down when we attempt to find the magnetic counterpart for the electric charge. While we find electric monopoles in the form of charged particles, single magnetic poles have never been seen in nature to occur spontaneously.

Dirac's theory pointed to something puzzling. It predicted the magnetic monopole, a north or south pole in isolation. Why does mathematics predict such strange behaviors? What are magnetic monopoles for? It seems completely crazy! In 1931, Dirac wrote: "one would be surprised if Nature had made no use of it." Since then, millions of dollars in research have poured in. Yet, as of 2019, more than eighty years since Dirac predicted magnetic monopoles, they remain elusive to science. In 1948, Dirac maintained: "Since electric charges are known to be quantized and no reason for this has yet been proposed apart from the existence of magnetic poles, we have here a reason for taking magnetic poles seriously."[193]

Tiller has a hunch about the monopole. It is astounding.

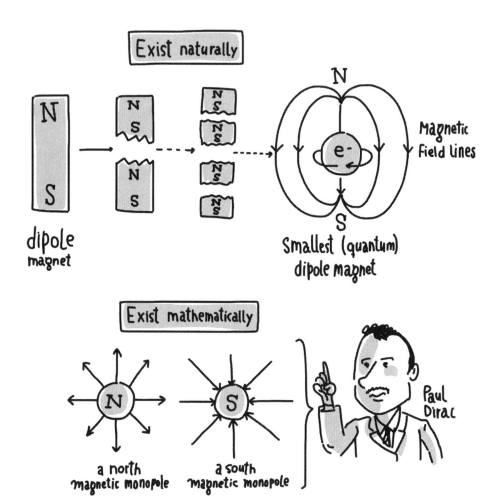

Exist naturally

dipole magnet

Magnetic Field Lines

Smallest (quantum) dipole magnet

Exist mathematically

a north magnetic monopole

a south magnetic monopole

Paul Dirac

[31]
"Space conditioning has a signature with magnetic monopole effects."
The Elusive Magnetic Monopole

"Might there be another novel and unique characteristic of a conditioned space in addition to oscillations?" Tiller asked himself. To investigate, let's say Tiller wants you to collaborate on his next experiment. Tiller wants to test the effect of a magnetic field on water pH in conditioned space versus in an ordinary unconditioned space. Moreover, he wants to investigate if a magnet's north pole versus its south pole will have distinct differences with respect to water pH. In other words, water pH could be a new and unique indicator of the quality of space. You are skeptical of his proposal for a couple of reasons:

> 1. Tiller wants to use an ordinary 100-Gauss magnet, the kind found on refrigerator doors. Gauss is a measure of the strength of magnetic fields. To put that into perspective, the Earth's magnetic field at its surface is about 0.5 Gauss. It is improbable for a field from a 100-Gauss magnet to have any effect on properties of liquid water like its pH in normal and familiar setup like a garage space.

> 2. Moreover, magnetic fields from the north pole and south pole are symmetric with respect to a magnet's orientation in space. It doesn't matter whether the water molecules are in a force field from a dipole magnet's

north pole or its south pole. Besides, it is a well-accept-
ed scientific observation that magnets are always dipolar, and magnetic monopoles, north or south, have never been observed to occur separately. Therefore, north
pole and south pole field effects would be identical; that
is, no change in water pH would be expected.

In your curiosity about Tiller's unusual theory, you both decide to test
the following hypothesis: a dipole magnet with its north pole or south
pole facing into a vessel containing water will have no effect on the
ionization of water and yield identical pH results for water.

You both agree to run the experiment in your respective garages
in Payson, Arizona. It's pretty straightforward. Tiller is setting up in
his garage down the road from yours. In your garage space, you set
up the water vessel and your benchtop Accumet pH meter with a resolution of ±0.001 pH units and fast response, high-performance glass
electrodes. Water temperature is measured using a SensorLink system with ±0.1 °C resolution. You calibrate the Accumet with custom
pH buffer solutions. Calculations from thermodynamic data predict
that the pH of ultrapure water in equilibrium with air at 25 °C is acidic with values about 5.60 to 5.70 because of dissolved carbon dioxide.
This value represents a kind of internal standard against which you
can compare measured experimental pH values.

You place your magnet with its north pole facing into the water
vessel. The data memory is set manually at one-minute intervals and
the digital recorder inputs pH data in real-time to a computer. Within
the first twenty minutes or so, you observe that the pH of the water
drops to an equilibrium value of 5.80, consistent with calculations,
and it settles there with minor wobbles of ± 0.01 units for the dura-

tion of the experiment. As predicted, in your garage, the north pole does not influence the water's ionization and pH balance.

Next, you repeat the experiment, this time with the south pole facing into the vessel containing water. Again, as expected, the water pH equilibrates with a few wobbles around a small range of 5.80 ± 0.01, identical to the data plot of the north pole. This isn't surprising because you know that the magnetic force field is symmetric: the magnet's thermodynamic potential is independent of its orientation in space. In other words, as already noted, we don't expect to detect any difference between the polarity of a north pole versus the polarity of a south pole. They should and do have exactly the same results on water pH, so nothing unexpected has happened.

You increase the strength of the magnet by switching the 100-Gauss magnet for a 500-Gauss magnet. You reason that a stronger magnet might improve outcomes and show differing effects of the north and south poles on the water pH in your garage. Unsurprisingly, the pH data with the stronger magnet are exactly identical to your earlier data and hover at expected equilibrium values. You are feeling pretty good. Thermodynamics has successfully predicted the results. All is in order.

You call Tiller to share the results of your respective experiments. He comes over with his water pH data. You look at it with puzzlement. The result from Tiller's garage space show that with the north pole, water pH decreases to become more acidic by 0.3 pH unit! His data with the south pole is similarly stunning: the water pH increases nearly 0.8 pH units above equilibrium. He also uses 100- and 500-Gauss magnets, and his results show, irrespective of the strength of the magnet, that the north pole lowers the water's pH, whereas the south pole increases it.[194]

You're baffled. How is it possible that a north pole and south pole have completely different water pH results? Impossible. Yet, there they are. Tiller's data are real. There is an obvious difficulty in explaining his results from a conventional perspective: any data that exhibits ΔpH that is different from equilibrium requires a physics wherein magnetic monopoles have an influence on material properties. But magnetic monopoles are thought not to exist spontaneously in nature.

You go to Tiller's garage. At first glance your eye passes right over the equipment, accepting the items as part of the experimental backdrop. But then something else registers in your awareness. There seems to be a vibrancy, a certain aliveness, a warmth in his garage. As you ponder the differences in results, it slowly dawns on you that you can *feel* something different in his garage. You recognize something of this, for the feeling is very strong. *You are standing in hallowed space.*

Tiller's results point to something extraordinary: there is more than one familiar dimension. There is the one we work in, sleep in, eat in, and where magnetic fields behave properly. But here is a different dimension that has been discovered through the intention research. Space is not a static, empty backdrop against which the theater of the universe plays out. It is a physical thing that can bend (in the presence of massive objects), ripple (called gravitational waves), or expand. Tiller is touching on a space attribute even more essential than these.

Tiller writes in *Conscious Acts of Creation: The Emergence of a New Physics:* "The key experiment revealing a fundamental change in the electromagnetic nature of the space associated with the conditioning process was a DC magnetic field polarity effect."[195] He is talking about a monopole effect, a singular signature of conditioned space. Science has been looking for more dimensions. What do the different spaces that Tiller describes—ordinary and conditioned—mean? What purpose could they serve in nature? The powerful concepts of symmetries in nature were indispensable in answering these questions.

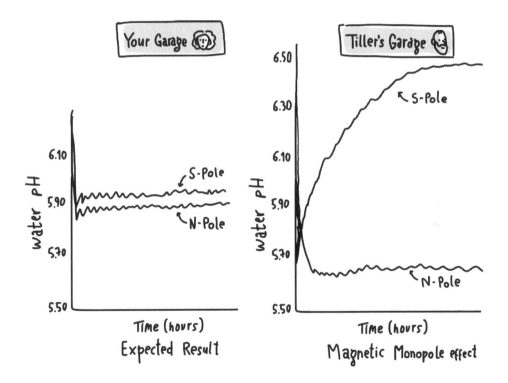

[32]
"A conditioned space means raising the symmetry of the physical vacuum's electromagnetic state."
Nature's Symmetries

Sometimes, deep insights into the working of nature are not the result of simply coming up with new equations, whether you are Dirac or Einstein. Instead, breakthroughs can come in realizing that things that appear different are, in fact, the same. Symmetry is important to understanding the significance of Tiller's "space-conditioning" and how that fits into the bridge. This section is a bit like a sightseeing tour of a vast and fascinating science.

Symmetry in this context means that something can be arranged in two different ways but nonetheless appear the same. If you take a square and turn it 90 degrees, it looks the same after the change as it did before the change. Reflect the square in a mirror, and again, the square looks the same. Translate (slide) it sideways without rotating, and the square looks the same. All these maneuvers—rotation, reflection, translation, lead to an invariance of the configurations of the square. The collection of all possible configurations is called a "group." Group theory is the mathematical language of symmetry.[196] A familiar type of symmetry is present in our own bodies. Specifically, the left and right halves of the human body are mirror images of each other, creating a two-sided or "bilateral" symmetry.

Crystallography was one of the first areas of science to benefit from group theory. Tiller is a world expert crystallographer. He has a deep working knowledge of the different types of crystals by considering the symmetries of the crystal's atomic lattice. Sodium chloride (ordinary table salt) forms an extremely regular cubic lattice. Diamonds and quartz are crystals that can be cut in a way that exactly divides two adjacent planes of atoms, often giving rise to spectacular optical clarity.

How do we know what the fundamental symmetries of space are? All directions in space appear to us to be equivalent. The laws of physics don't know the difference between up and down, forward and backward, or sideways. Space has fields generated by subatomic particles, such as electron fields formed by electrons, Higgs boson fields formed by Higgs bosons, and so on. Gauge theory is a mathematical theory used to describe subatomic particles and their associated wave fields. Gauge symmetry is the observation that you can redefine the fields or particles in terms of each other in such a way that the laws remain the same. This is called "gauge invariance" and gives the theory a certain symmetry.[197]

Mathematician Ian Stewart, in his book *Why Beauty Is Truth: A History of Symmetry,* illustrates the last point, defining fields and particles in terms of each other, with the so-called "currency rule."[198]

Suppose that you (particle) are traveling in another country, let's call it Duplicatia, and you need money. The Duplicatian currency is the "drueble" and the exchange rate is two druebles to the dollar. You notice a simple and obvious rule for translating dollars into druebles. Namely, everything costs twice as many druebles as you would expect to pay in dollars.

This is a kind of symmetry. The "laws" of commercial transactions are unchanged if you double all the numbers. To compensate for the numerical difference, though, you pay in drueble currency, not in dollars. This "invariance under the change of monetary scale" is a global symmetry of the rules for commercial transactions. If you make the same change throughout, the rules are invariant.

Just across the border, in neighboring Triplicatia, the local currency is the "troodle" and it is valued at *three* to the dollar. When you take a day trip to Triplicatia, the corresponding symmetry requires all the sums to be multiplied by three. Again, the laws of commerce remain invariant.

Now we have a "symmetry" that differs from one place to another. In Duplicatia, it is multiplied by two. In Triplicatia, it is multiplied by three. You would not be surprised to find that on visiting Quadlicatia, the corresponding multiple is four. These symmetry operations can be applied simultaneously, but each is valid only in the corresponding country. The laws of commerce are still invariant, but only if you interpret the numbers according to the correct local currency.

This local rescaling of currency transactions is a gauge symmetry of the laws of commerce. In principle, the exchange rate could be different at every point of space and time, but the laws would still be invariant provided you interpreted all transactions in terms of the local value of the "currency field."

Back to physics. Like exchange rates applied to currencies, gauge transforms can be applied mathematically and geometrically to quantum fields, making the models easier to analyze.[199] The currencies relate to vector potentials in magnetic fields. When you measure force fields of elementary particles, you discover that the conservation law holds. Just as we don't suddenly have extra cash in Duplicatia, we also don't suddenly have extra energy. The force fields give shape and structure to the universe of particles; they provide the invisible skeleton. For every conservation law, there is a symmetry. For every symmetry, there is a force field. For every force field, there is a conservation law.[200]

This brings us to the good old familiar field: electromagnetic. The classical theory of the electromagnetic field, proposed by Scottish physicist James Clerk Maxwell in 1864, is the prototype of gauge theories. In Maxwell's theory, the basic field variables are the electric and magnetic field strengths, which may be described in terms of auxiliary variables (e.g., the vector potentials).[201] The gauge transformations in this theory change the values of those potentials without changing the electric and magnetic fields. This gauge invariance is preserved in the modern theory of electromagnetism called quantum electrodynamics (QED).[202] The concept of gauge invariance is seen by physicists as fundamental to understanding classical and particle physics.

Tiller uses the shorthand notation of gauge theory. For example, the electromagnetic field in ordinary space is U(1) gauge. Higher order than U(1) is SU(2) gauge, which signifies rotations in 3D space and governs the interaction between electromagnetism and the weak nuclear force. The SU(2) gauge is the state where both electrical charges and magnetic fields coexist. Higher order still is the gauge SU(3), which governs "quantum chromodynamics," the underlying theory of the strong nuclear force. While the letters are from group theory notation, the numbers refer to how many independent phase angles exist in that particular gauge state. There are many gauge states higher than SU(3), up to any SU[n]. Tiller's working hypothesis is that the IHD information "lifts" space, a process he calls "conditioning," from the familiar electromagnetic U(1) gauge to the higher level of SU(2) gauge. A space at SU(2) gauge can operate in the physical vacuum.

As a medium, space and its symmetries control the dynamics of the physical interactions of matter. Symmetry, ultimately, is a tool that lets us not only figure out the rules but also figure out why those rules work.[203] So, what does this all mean? The world of electromagnetism, which we know well, is not the only reality. Nature has more in store.

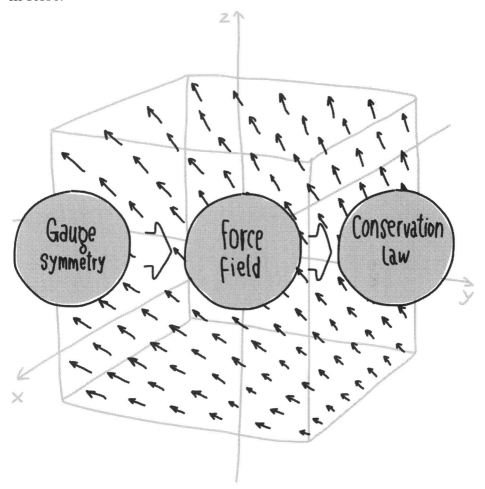

[33]
"Space conditioning requires a new type of reference frame than just space-time for viewing nature."
Beyond Spacetime: Dual Realities

Tiller's moonshot strategy of using an IHD to investigate intention was rewarded by the discovery of behavior in another dimension of space, not only otherworldly nondispersive "wave" behavior but, remarkably, magnetic monopole effects. His experimental evidence points to the necessity for a new frame of reference that includes more dimensions than the familiar spacetime. Tiller isn't the first to suggest more dimensions. The idea that nature has more than four dimensions has long been on the mind of physicists, as it would help answer many deep questions about the workings of the universe. "Superstring theory" is one such current hot topic, but it has proved diabolically difficult to perform experiments on, making it unfalsifiable. Tiller sought a concrete, testable theory.

Tiller calls the familiar four-dimensional world of matter (all elementary particles) and its governing forces such as electromagnetism and gravity "direct space," or "D-space." This is the standard model at U(1). Tiller's data points to a second dimension having magnetic wave information characteristics but not material stuff: the physical vacuum at SU(2) gauge symmetry. Tiller calls the SU(2) "reciprocal space" or "R-space." Keep in mind, when we talk about D-space, it is the familiar U(1) gauge, and when talking about R-space, it is the otherworldly SU(2) gauge.

Now take a deep breath. Relax. It's all a little technical, but it'll make sense. You may find me repeating some notions, but it is intentional so that you become familiar with new concepts. Remember, we are at the cutting edge of research, and we need new terms to describe never-before-directly-observed features of nature.

Tiller gives a mathematical relationship between D-space and R-space with Fourier transform geometry. You can calculate and show that R-space is of a *negative* energy state of the Dirac sea and comprises the physical vacuum; this is the nondispersive medium. Remember, Dirac chose an arbitrary starting point for the vacuum as "negative energy" states. The waveforms in R-space control the position, velocity, and locus of particles in the "now" of D-space. In other words, the R-space's pilot waves guide D-space particles and matter such as electrons. Tiller's model corresponds to the familiar wave-particle duality of French physicist Louis de Broglie.[204] At the great physics conference in Solvay in 1927, it was de Broglie who first proposed an alternative theory that imagined particles riding on "pilot waves."[205] The waves in Tiller's model are superluminal, faster than the speed of light, and have a magnetic nature.

Another special relationship between D-space and R-space is mirror symmetry. If you reflect, say, your home in a mirror, you can plot each point from its original D-space location to its matching mirror-image location in R-space. The twist here is that R-space is a reciprocal variation of D-space. In mathematics, a reciprocal variation is a procedure that "reverses" another function.[206] When you take data points of your home—its height, depth, and length—and apply a reciprocal function, you're taking 1/height, 1/depth, and 1/length. The beautiful thing is that if you plot all the D-space points of your home on a graph, and then, all the reciprocal function points for R-space, you will get a mirror-like symmetry. It's a natural consequence of reciprocal functions. You can also go in reverse from any point in R-space to its associate in D-space. Your home isn't the Taj Mahal with its admirable reflective mirror symmetry. But on a graph, your home emerges perfectly from R-space with its equivalent, corresponding mirror symmetry in D-space.

The mirror exists. Look around you . . . everything and every place in the "real" world of D-space has its twin in the mirror world of R-space. The virtual R-space is a high-resolution blueprint of information overlaying your world: the book you're holding, the chair you're sitting on, the lamp on your desk, the street outside your window, the home across the street.

Looking at the reciprocal variation more closely, we can see that as the denominator increases (points in D-space), the R-space becomes smaller and—wait, it gets crazy here—reaches infinity! Let's say the distance from the ground to the roof of your home (D-space) is X meters. If you calculate $1/X$ meters, then you can see that the result for R-space of your home is small. You can't "see" the R-space aspect of your home, but you can calculate it. The spatially far apart distance between the ground and the roof becomes tiny in R-space.

Are you seeing what I am seeing? Spatially, points in R-space are very close. As time in D-space increases, then its inverse, $1/\text{time}$, means that in R-space, you can reach infinity! Timelessness! The math of infinity seems, to me, to collide with logic and reason. But history shows us that the mathematicians pursued it and developed very useful math. Tiller says the seat of all subtle energies functions at this vacuum level of nature, that is, SU(2). The bridge between subtle energies of R-space and the physical D-space is the magnetic vector potential. This property, this connection, sheds light on psychoenergetic capabilities such as remote viewing.

Science has struggled to unify weird quantum behaviors. It's more complex when we consider human capabilities like remote viewing and action-from-a-distance. With the dual D-space and R-space, so much is dispensed with: the whole cumbersome machinery of strings, superstrings, and so on. In their place, Tiller provides raw data that gives us insights and a new way to unify different aspects of our amazing universe.

But what does all this mean for you and me? Are these extra dimensions good for something other than remote viewing and access to regions of space we can't normally get to? Can R-space be good for something more practical? Look at it this way: What if this empty space had energy to it, like a glow or a low hum, even if it has no matter?[207]

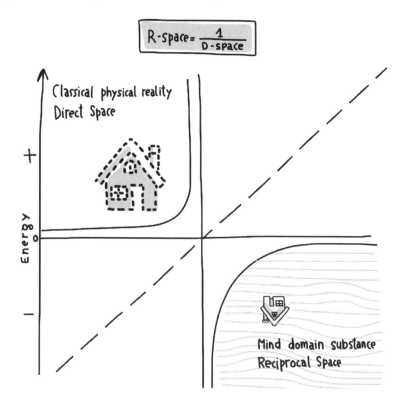

[34]
"There is higher thermodynamic free energy available in conditioned space."
Thermodynamics of a Conditioned Space

We can now reconsider the water and its unaccountable shift in pH against equilibrium. Physicists are trained to look for equilibrium, which is another way of saying: "When you change one thing, how do other things respond? Where do things settle once all interactions have occurred?"

To change water pH, some energy is needed to bring about a reaction, such as changes in ionic bonds. What do we mean by "the energy needed"? We have to get a little bit technical here and introduce the common currency in talking about the energies of interactions of ions. Energy in this context is usually described with the *energy* unit *electron volt* (symbol: eV) which is a measure known as "joules"—not to be confused with the electric potential which is familiar to us as "voltage."[208] An example of different units, length has two possible units: metric (meters) and imperial (inches). We can use either unit to measure length and switch between the them. The same rule is true of joules and electron volts.

If we jolt water molecules with a source of energy (ΔG) of about 10 eV, it can cause a chemical reaction to occur in D-space. This outcome is well established by physics and chemistry. One of the most practical results of Tiller's experimental work is that he can now quantitatively measure the excess ΔG relative to the known values expected in D-space. By means of thermodynamic equations, he calculates the amount of excess energy needed to create more hydrogen ions (H^+) in his water target and reach a new equilibrium pH value. The results of his calculations show that new factors are necessary to add to the temperature, pressure, volume—those familiar things—and the excess ΔG necessary to tilt the equilibrium balance is *from the SU(2) gauge level of R-space.*

The foregoing means that the measured water pH is a combination of equilibrium expected pH (as a result of D-space effects) plus additional pH change (as a result of R-space effects). Calculating the extra energy, or the R-space contribution, is straightforward:

$$\text{Measured water } \Delta pH \text{ actual} =$$
$$\Delta pH \text{ D-space (expected)} + \Delta pH \text{ R-space contribution}$$

$$\Delta pH \text{ R-space contribution} =$$
$$\text{Measured water } \Delta pH \text{ actual} - \Delta pH \text{ D-space (expected)}$$

If you have a ΔpH of one unit in D-space (say, from a pH of 5.6 to a pH of 6.6) it is equivalent to the internal energy change of an atom that is heated by 300°C! This is a substantial amount of energy in thermal terms. Tiller converted the effective temperature change to its thermodynamic energy equivalent of milli-electron volts (meV).

He thereby established a new and original thermodynamic term for the R-space aspect of his lab which he designated as ΔG^{*}_{H+}. All water pH measurements could be mathematically scaled to this newly described standard. A one-unit increase in water pH is equivalent to a free energy ΔG^{*}_{H+} of 24.5 meV.[209] A remarkable follow-on from this is that Tiller now could quantify, put a number as an indicator of the degree of conditioned space, with ΔG^{*}_{H+}.

Tiller uses the term "magnetoelectric" for the subtle energy effects of intention. This is drawn from an accepted, albeit limited, vocabulary that necessarily seems to repeat itself. "Magnetoelectric" is an expansion of the electromagnetic potential by the addition of a magnetic energy term (itself the product of a magnetic charge and a magnetic potential).[210] The way I remember magnetoelectric is with the letters "ME." This new thermodynamic energy contribution arises from the proposed existence of heretofore experimentally inaccessible magnetic information wave signatures in a "conditioned" space.

Another way to put it: lifting the experimental space from D-space to R-space via the IHD increases the thermodynamic free energy of that space. We know from the science of thermodynamics, processes in nature flow from higher thermodynamic free energy states to lower thermodynamic free energy states. The ΔpH of water is an indicator of the magnitude of the conditioning of a space.

The change in material properties is energy flowing from a high source to low one doing work. It's not so different from a car rolling down a hill or the pressure cooker's shrill whistle to tell you dinner is ready. Tiller's task was to find out what parameters changed in the second law of thermodynamics to contribute to ΔG^*_{H+}, which I will henceforth label as ΔG^*_{pH}.

From the general equation, we can begin to deduce to what degree the various terms changed:

$$\Delta G^*_{pH} = PV + E - TS$$

The pressure (P) or the volume (V) of the laboratory did not change. The internal energy (E) and temperature (T) remain constant (except for the oscillations already described), and the lab is not burning up at 300°C. Tiller says: "There was just one term, S. The change is entropic."

In plain old-fashioned physics, intention does not counter the laws of thermodynamics. The intention is a source of information that is connected quantitatively to entropy. An increase in *new* information equals a reduction in entropy, in this case of the lab space. Human intention influences or "coheres" the vacuum state to a more ordered state. A reduction in entropy—negentropy—contributes to Gibbs free energy.

There is a connection between D-space and R-space. It's a question of degree, from no connectivity, zero, to complete connectivity, one. If space is conditioned, partially or wholly, it is at a higher thermodynamic free energy, which has power to make things happen.

Tiller continues: "Our work implies that if you had a device that could connect U(1) and SU(2), it could do useful work! It's a thermodynamic 'pump.' That is what thermodynamics is all about!"

The important point about Tiller's work is that he took thermodynamics that had been measured in the laboratory and extrapolated it to new conditions to show how intention works. He showed that thermodynamics and entropy are experimentally observable and measurable factors in intention research. He takes the world of psychoenergetic science and bridges it with thermodynamics. Not only that, he puts a number on it. Can you think of a better example of the power of the principle of universality?

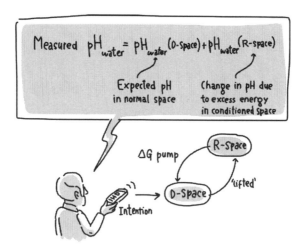

[35]
"There is another communication channel in nature. The R-space is the medium whereby information is transferred. It is information entanglement."
Macroscopic Informational Entanglement in Space and Time

From 2000 to 2005, Tiller teamed up with physicists in Baltimore and Bethesda, Maryland, as well as in London, Milan, and Berlin to replicate the water pH experiments.[211] Tiller was keen to collaborate with other scientists. With collaboration from these scientists, the lab setup spread from the East Coast of the US to Europe. Some labs were designated as control sites without any devices. For example, the laboratory in Milan did not have an IHD when the Italian physicists joined the protocol. Then something curious happened.

The scientists in Milan were setting up their tabletop kit with the sealed water vessel, digital pH meter, and all the equipment that Tiller used to exact specifications. Physically, they were 5,794 miles from Arizona, where Tiller was busy in his lab in Payson. Without any IHD, the pH of the water in the sealed vessel began to behave anomalously. They contacted Tiller. He realized that there was connectivity or, to use a better term, *entanglement* between sites. The ΔpH information can be readily "transferred" from Payson to Milan via R-space. It cannot happen via D-space. The same thing occurred with the control sites in Baltimore and Bethesda.

In their paper "Toward General Experimentation and Discovery in Conditioned Laboratory Spaces. Part IV: Macroscopic Information Entanglement Between Sites 6000 Miles Apart," Tiller and his co-authors noted that what was particularly striking about the results of these experiments is that the anomalous effects seem to be independent of how far away the other lab is, spatially.[212] These unusual effects show that intention's ability to generate information can affect the physical world is real and can be demonstrated under controlled, scientific conditions.

This mechanism of long-range, macroscopic-scale information entanglement distinguishes R-space. Tiller postulates that this information transfer process is related to magnetic monopole behavior that generates an entirely *new type of field* in human experience. Without the Faraday cage, in the early target experiments, the UED controls were lost because of entanglement in R-space. R-space sets up information entanglement between IHD sites and control sites located a few miles away, to nearly six thousand miles away. A premise we hold from the second law of thermodynamics asserts that a system autonomously tending to an organized state cannot be closed and separate. We must consider the possibility that, in an open system such as that Tiller's colleagues in US and Europe created, nature can "import" organization into one region from another via R-space.

Tiller makes a significant point: in space with electromagnetic fields, the important qualities of interest are *vectors*. Vector is a math concept used to describe the rate of change at each point in a field. For a vector system of multiple parts, such as the entire universe, there is always an *information entanglement* between the parts because they are never totally isolated from each other. This is a description of nature. We cannot prove it. However, as with the first law of thermodynamics of energy conservation, mathematics shows that information entanglement effects must be accounted for to offer a complete description of physical observations.

Biologist Lyall Watson writes on this point: "We are normally slow to make direct connections between physical events and the people involved because of a mindset which pervades science and common sense.[213] It is reinforced by the language we use to describe events." We say: "A physicist in Milan looked at water pH." Simple enough on the surface, but the syntax conceals a host of presuppositions. The familiar sequence of subject-verb-object implies that the subject, a physicist in Milan, is a separate entity in whom the action of "looking" both occurs and is confined. The object—water—is set apart in space as another separate entity, equally fixed in its nature, following its own set of rules.

But if the new Tiller physics is right, then this view is simplistic and misleading because it is incomplete. What we should be saying about the events in Milan is: "Observations took place in connected actions and operations involving the entities we describe as a 'physicist in Milan' and 'water.'" That is excessively cumbersome, but it comes closer to the truth, which is that things are elaborately connected, and it is impossible ever to be totally isolated and objective.

Again, Tiller's "technical" terminology for information entanglement is the "Granny effect." Granny's information reaches you wherever you are in space and time. You receive it via the R-space component! Isn't nature cool? Like your Granny.

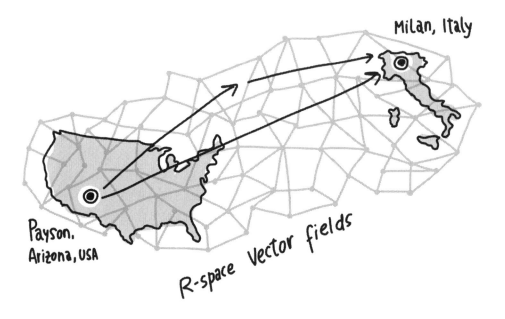

Milan, Italy

Payson,
Arizona, USA

R-space Vector fields

[36]
"I postulate a new particle, deltron, that connects direct-space with reciprocal-space."
What's in a Name: Deltrons[214]

Tiller speaks: "Thy Will be Done." We are now entering our favorite realm. The realm beyond a dense world of computers and meters, thermometers and graphs that becomes fuzzy, its outline merely granular. Anyone coming into the lab would have seen Tiller and three graduate students sitting in meditative silence. But we deltrons are not really in that room. In truth, we have long departed into ourselves. We departed the subluminal D-space universe. Accelerating faster than the speed of light, the jam-packed Higgs boson and its field cannot stop us, for we have no mass. Faster than the protons and neutrons hugging tightly, tightly the strong force binding them securely in an atom's nucleus. That's all they know. That's their universe, but it's not ours. We hear the cries of quarks, the fundamental building blocks of matter beckoning us to join them. We know better. Our velocity breezes past 186,000 miles per second. We overtake photons carrying light. We don't let that affect us. We like to keep moving. Emotions of joy, elation, and possibility culminate in our hearts and we swoop faster still, quickening. Whoosh!

Suddenly, we tunnel from D-space into R-space and find ourselves rotating, levitating splendidly with perfect symmetry in wave-like formations of the negative Dirac sea. There is no gravity in our reciprocal universe. People don't see us. They think of us, if they know about us at all, as a speck of void. The D-space world casts but a faint shadow onto our abode in the R-space field. No-where and no-time, for we are beyond both, our existence arising in the information field of super-consciousness of the Cosmic Mind. Magnetic monopoles wink in and out of existence in topological super-space contours.

As we expand in numbers, we pump the D-space, laser-like, with excess thermodynamic energy exciting the electrons above ground state. The notion of an intelligent Earth nourished in its turn by an intelligent system of energy is fulfilled. Thy Will be Done.

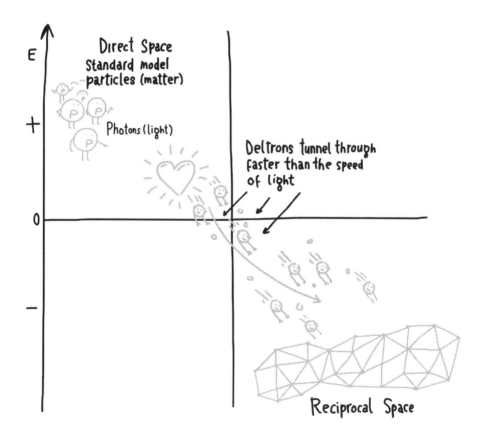

[37]
"Humans create field effects."
Love My Garage

The field is like a canvas, but unlike a flat canvas it interacts with the physical vacuum and shapes the stuff in it. There are field effects present in every part of life's marvelous machinery, and I suspect that one of the most potent of these is the capacity we have to influence the world around us directly. I believe that it is possible for an idea, particularly one that is strongly housed at an unconscious level, to manifest its own independent physical reality.

In the imprinting process, emotion is a crucial ingredient. Pumped up, it creates a field in the lab space, conditioning it. Subjectively at least, more emotion seems to imprint the IHD robustly. The IHD, like a laser, continues to pump a coherent beam of information generated by humans into the space where it is deployed. Emotion in the larger perspective is informational, but not in a Shannon bit sense. To illustrate the importance of emotions, Tiller gives an example of what he calls "the garage inventor effect."[215]

Suppose there is a man, a hobbyist, who works in his garage after dinner on his latest invention. He has an idea for creating a machine for electric power conversion with greater than 100 percent efficiency. He wants to develop a prototype that demonstrates his idea.

For several years, this man works most nights in his garage designing his invention. One evening, he feels certain that he has finally accomplished this "over unity" energy conversion apparatus. Excited, the next evening he calls in a small group of his best friends to demonstrate his success and show them how he accounted for all the critical technical factors relevant to the invention. After pondering all the related issues, the group concludes that he has achieved a great new discovery.

Collectively, they decide to start a new business to profit from this new invention and also help the world solve its energy crisis. One member of the group suggests they take the apparatus and all the measurement equipment to a company in the next town that performs independent verification for a fee. All agree that this is a good idea and carefully pack up the equipment and drive it to the next town for independent replication.

After a month, the testing information comes back. To the group's great disappointment, it indicates the apparatus only achieves normal efficiency. This doesn't make sense because the testing company used precisely the same meticulous measuring procedures as did the inventor with their own high-grade measuring equipment. Even using the inventor's measurement equipment, they still achieved only standard results. How can these two very different results be true? Surely, all factors were accounted for.

Actually, all the relevant factors in the replication experiment were not the same. In the garage inventor's case, his strong desire, sustained for years, pumped deltrons slowly into the garage space via his subtle energy pump, so he gradually conditioned his garage from D-space to R-space. On the other hand, we can assume that the testing company's experimental space was at D-space, without mimicking the inventor's strong desire.

The important point to conclude from this example is that the level of "space conditioning" is a key part of the inventor's new apparatus, and it must be present with the apparatus for it to exhibit supernormal behavior. In this supernormal state, the apparatus draws in energy from the magnetic information wave level of R-space in nature. From the perspective of D-space reality, the R-space contribution takes it "over the top" to greater than 100 percent efficiency.

The garage inventor example illustrates something of the importance of the unacknowledged field effects of the locations where events occur. It is important to recognize that sustained human intention, whether unconscious or conscious, flavored by strong desire, can significantly raise the electromagnetic gauge symmetry state of a workspace. When you and I sit down and work, we become like a magnetized rod that attracts iron filings. Ideas come. Insights accrete. Power concentrates around us.[216] Our subtle energies pump and fields are created, which means dealing with capabilities that are closer to R-space. It's not enough to just talk about physical things. Fields are like codes of grammar describing interactions and events. In these situations, we cease to speak of the physical world as if it were made of things only.

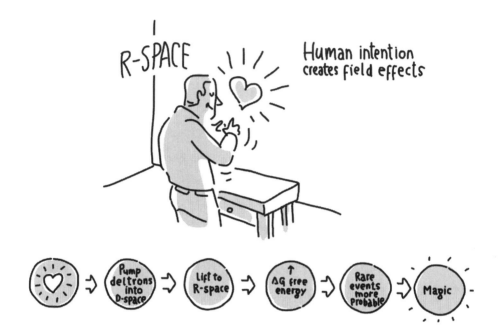

[38]
"The term 'zero-point energy' is misunderstood by the general public to mean something to do with consciousness.'."
The Big Freeze

Popular notions about the science of consciousness are jam-packed with words such as "frequency," "vibration," "matrix," "quantum," and my all-time favorite, "zero-point energy." This is a buzzword soup, an indecipherable mix of random terms and phrases. Clearly, such a situation should send us back to the first principles of physics to clarify the point. In fact, Tiller tells me: "Go to the source."

Since zero-point energy is so pervasive in discussions around consciousness, and to clear up my own confusion, I sought the original meaning of this concept. I took Albert Einstein's famous strategy of performing a hypothetical experiment, a *Gedankenexperiment,* which means literally a "thought experiment," for my exercise.

From classical thermodynamics, I knew that the notion of temperature is directly related to the amount of kinetic energy associated with a sample material; in other words, how fast the atoms that make up the material are moving or jiggling about. The existence of an absolute zero of temperature is then easy to understand; it is the state where particles stop moving completely and have zero kinetic energy. Clearly, no lower temperature is possible.

I wanted to test whether, as the temperature is reduced to absolute zero, atoms in my test material, sodium gas, came to a complete rest and ceased moving. This is my hypothetical point. So, I got into my *Gedankenexperiment* lab, located in Bemidji, Minnesota. When

I conducted my experiment, it was winter and the polar vortex had descended into the Midwest, giving me a perspective of what cold feels like. The outside temperature was a teeth-chattering minus 40 °C (-40 °F) with a wind chill of -65 °C (-85 °F).[217] In my thought lab, it was about to get a whole lot colder.

Insofar as there is a "scientific" scale for temperature, I used what physicists call the Kelvin scale. Named after William Thomson, also known as Lord Kelvin, one of the founders of thermodynamics, this scale effectively takes the Celsius temperature scale and shifts it. Instead of water freezing at 0 °C, it does so at 273 K, and it boils at 373 K (equivalent to 100 °C). The zero in the Kelvin scale is taken to be absolute zero—and it is cold! It measures -273.16 °C.

To begin cooling my sodium gas, I bypassed liquid nitrogen, which at 77 K (-196 °C) is too warm for my purpose. However, it is possible to cool a mixture of liquid helium-3 and helium-4 to a few thousandths of a kelvin. Instead, I proceeded (imagining I have great research funding) to use cleverer technology, as scientists did in 2003 at the Massachusetts Institute of Technology, using laser infrared light to slow down and thereby cool fast-moving atomic particles.[218] In my mind, I could "see" the sodium atoms at room temperature moving at the speed of a jet airplane and slowing down with each laser pulse in my *Gedankenexperiment.*

I got my equipment—the all-essential thermometer—and immediately came to a first hurdle. How could I be certain that I had reached absolute zero? First of all, any thermometer that was not itself at absolute zero would add heat and ruin the experiment. Second, it is hard to measure temperature at such low energies, where other effects, such as superconductivity and quantum mechanics, intervene and affect the motions and states of the atoms. I can never know for sure that I have gotten there, but I come very close, within a fraction of a degree Kelvin.

The second hurdle was a big one. At atomic levels, I came upon the fundamental constraint of physics—a physical limit, namely, the Heisenberg principle.[219] The German physicist Werner Heisenberg determined in 1927 that it is impossible to learn both the position and the momentum of a particle to a high degree of accuracy. If the position is known perfectly, then the momentum is completely unknown and vice versa. That's why near absolute zero, sodium particles must still be jittering about. If they were at a complete standstill, the momentum and position would both be known precisely and simultaneously, violating the uncertainty principle. This is one of the weird ambiguities of the subatomic world. I'd hit a wall.

I compiled the results from my *Gedankenexperiment* for an international scientific conference attended by Nobel Laureates Arno Penzias and Robert Wilson, who know a thing or two about absolute zero temperature. They determined the background radiation temperature of space at a value of 3.5 K.[220] I informed them that absolute zero itself had not been reached in my laboratory because no thermometer could measure it. Even with near-absolute zero, the hypothesis was shown to be incorrect. The motions of sodium atoms continue even with super-cooling and never vanish due to the uncertainty principle of quantum mechanics. I further advised the conference attendees that absolute zero is an abstract idea. To suck out all the energy, every last bit of it, and achieve zero energy and absolute zero temperature would take the age of the universe to accomplish.[221]

Back to the popular notion that consciousness is somehow related to zero-point energy. Zero-point energy is about a physical boundary. Consciousness research, on the other hand, whether brain science or

Tillerian physics, is at room temperature. I had to admit it does not hold up. Another fundamental issue is that my *Gedankenexperiment* lab is in D-space. I am seeing "usual" physical behavior at extreme temperature conditions. This is also the case for other physics labs conducting zero-point energy research. Zero-point isn't anything to do with consciousness.

I reported to Tiller following my thought experiment. Chuckling, he said: "The term zero-point energy is misunderstood to mean something to do with consciousness. This error gets in the way of true understanding. The physics of the zero-point energy is not pointing to a 'matrix.' Eventually people will get it."

I got it.

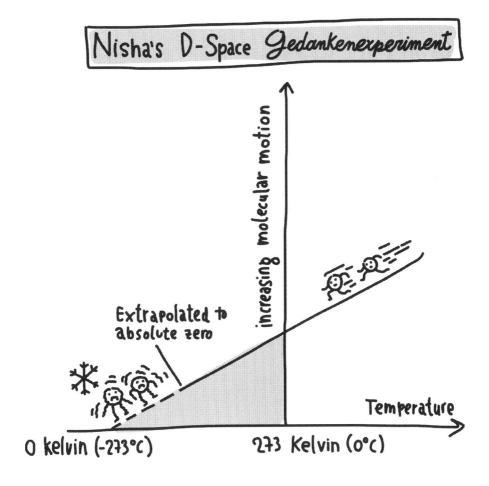

Strongly developed egotistic [intellectual] consciousness is a barrier, but at the same time it is a power. The barrier can be mastered, and the power retained. Highly developed capacity in relative knowledge is not to be scorned. Many genuinely Illumined Men have not seen clearly with respect to this point. The result is that while such men have made the Crossing for Themselves, they have left poor bridges for others. It is this bridge-building that is the really important work.

—Franklin Merrell-Wolff

in *Pathways through to Space: An Experiential Journal* [222]

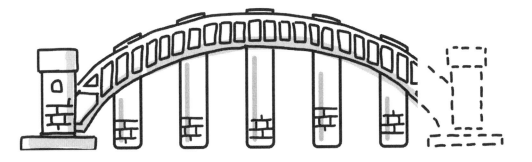

BRIDGE PILLAR 6:
Subtle Energy and Information Medicine for the Twenty-First Century: Subluminal and Superluminal Bridge Together.

Jesus replied: "Love the Lord your God with all your heart and with all your soul and with all your mind. This is the first and greatest commandment. And the second is like it: Love your neighbor as yourself. All the Law and the Prophets hang on these two commandments."

–MATTHEW 22: 36–40

We're not stuck in distance–time the way our orthodox science thinks we are, and our orthodox medicine thinks we are.
If we give what I'm saying (meaning) about this other aspect of nature that we're one with, then we will grow into it and become it, and it will fuel us for the great adventure ahead.

–WILLIAM A. TILLER[223]

[39]
"The acupuncture system is the energy pump in the human body."
Your Power Is Within You

Since the time you were a tiny babe, you have sent energy from an inner fountain in your body through to your nerves, to your muscles and organs for work. Whenever you have done so, you have not been conscious of the source of subtle magnetoelectric energy or the fact that it was arriving at its destination. Below the surface of your skin lie energetic systems that can't be understood with the eyes alone. The most skilled anatomists carefully dissect and examine the body's tissues and come up empty.

When he measured the conditioned lab space and revealed the astonishing nested harmonics, Tiller asked an important question: "Might there be some system in our bodies that is at a higher gauge symmetry state? Something we are born with? Because if there is, then that can 'pump' what we call life. It would make synapses work, make the brain cells go, and pump the heart! All vital processes of the atoms-molecules in our cells would run. Remember, all of life, and [that] includes human life, is based upon a thermodynamic potential driving force. This force, this potential, drives all the kinetic processes and transformations in the cells of our bodies." Tiller's dual-space theory finds one of its grandest expressions in the human body!

To check his theory, he did a simple test. Using a bar magnet (dipole) as a probe, Tiller proceeded to test various muscle groups response to monopoles by placing the south pole close, within one centimeter of the skin surface and examined the muscle strength with kinesiology. He found the south pole strengthens muscles, while the north pole weakens them. The body "knows" a north pole versus a south pole, meaning there is a symmetry, similar to the physical vacuum gauge state, already within your body. Tiller pointed out: "It is not the material stuff of the atoms and molecules of the nerves or muscle that is responding. It cannot be a U(1) gauge response. Monopole effects strongly indicate that the human body has a system already at a higher gauge symmetry, or SU(2)."[224]

Questions naturally arise about what Tiller's observations mean for clinical medicine. This being outside of my formal education, I turned to two resources to discover more. First, I searched the National Library of Medicine of the National Institute of Health. I would *like* to report that medical science has performed clinical trials to test the hypothesis of magnetic monopole effects in people in health and disease. But it has not done so. There have been sporadic efforts to investigate the effects of magnets on biologic systems, but these studies have dissipated as time went on.

Luckily, I was rewarded with an editorial by Richard Niemtzow, MD, PhD, MPH, in the journal *Medical Acupuncture* titled "Acupuncture and Magnets: Is There a Clinical Role?"[225] He reports that magnets are being used to reinforce the therapeutic benefit of acupuncture in the Veterans Health Administration system. He goes on to describe the work of Isaac Goiz Duràn, MD, and Richard Broeringmeyer, MD, DC, PhD, HMD, stating: ". . . A significant number of diseases (presence of viruses, bacteria, fungi, parasites, toxins, and cancers) cause changes in the pH balance in the body. In short, placing N and S poles of two magnets, respectively, in a specific manner causes elimination of the pathogen and restoration of the body's pH balance, resulting in healing."[226]

In the same issue of *Medical Acupuncture,* the original article "Biomagnetic Pair Therapy and Typhoid Fever: A Pilot Study," by Bryan L. Frank, MD, reported on the magnet therapy being used to treat typhoid fever in rural Kenya.[227] Muscle testing was first used to energetically identify organs and tissues out of normal polarity by strength of the deltoid muscle or thumb and an opposing finger (see Appendix 2).[228] Then magnets were used to treat the unbalanced organs. All the people with typhoid reported improvement, and, on retesting, most of them showed clearing of *Salmonella typhi,* the bacteria that causes typhoid fever. Typhoid fever is serious and prevalent in rural populations. That a simple strategy using magnets worked is, to my mind (and I'm from Kenya), astonishing.

Tiller, with his simple curiosity, had found that north poles and south poles have different effects on water pH in his conditioned Payson laboratory. His curiosity led him to test the human body's response to magnets. Medical research is in the very early stages of magnet therapy, and the preliminary reports point to possibilities that could have profound implications for future medicine. *Yowza.* Tiller's basic observations are ahead of medical science.

Muscle testing, initially presented by chiropractic George Goodheart in 1964, has been shown to have clinical utility by many respected clinicians, including Dr. John Diamond. Information, whether in chemical, verbal, nonverbal, or virtually any form an examiner wants to test, can be tested with muscle strength in an individual. My brain went into overdrive. I can think of more than a dozen rheumatic diseases that could benefit from these effects, and fibromyalgia tops the list.

What should we conclude from this? My second resource, the second edition of *Bioelectromagnetic and Subtle Energy Medicine,*

edited by Paul J. Rosch, MD, gives the prediction of orthopedic surgeon and proponent of bioelectric medicine, the late C. Andrew L.
Bassett.[229] Bassett's view was that, in the diseases to come, it was safe
to predict that bioelectromagnetics would assume a therapeutic importance equal to or greater than that of pharmacology and surgery
today. With proper interdisciplinary effort, significant inroads can be
made in controlling the ravages of cancer, some forms of heart disease, arthritis, hormonal disorders, and neurologic scourges such as
Alzheimer's disease, spinal-cord injury, and multiple sclerosis. As Dr.
Niemtzow noted, this prediction was not "pie-in-the sky." Pilot studies and biologic mechanisms already described in primordial terms
form a rational basis for such a statement.[230]

What does it mean for you? Bottom line, your body has within
it a higher energy system. Your body has U(1), which is the "material stuff" of the body, and SU(2), the acupuncture system pumping qi
(subtle energy to the nerves and cells). Higher still, as Tiller postulates, is the chakra system at SU(3). Not only humans but probably all
vertebrates have a qi pump providing "life."

Just as moving a magnet generates an electric current, so your
acupuncture system, being magnetoelectric—which I term "ME," creates electrical currents when stimulated with an acupuncture needle
or with tai chi. Like a process of a step-down transformer, energy
flows from your SU(2) level down to the levels where your nerve cells
run, your digestive juices and enzymes are powered up, and your
brain cells take in thought. Energy flow through a system works to
organize that system. We cannot see these energy superhighways,
but we can measure the resulting electric currents in muscle or brain
tissue with electromyography (EMG) and electroencephalography
(EEG), respectively.

You can significantly enhance the magnitude and qualities of the energies and information flowing in your acupuncture meridian and chakra systems. Practices like directed intention, meditation, yoga, qigong, and tai chi can significantly strengthen and broaden the qi flows, which in turn enhance the electrical potential in your cells.[231] The acupuncture meridian system is the bridge to the superluminal domain—faster than the speed of light! We cannot hope to visually see this in biomedicine; we don't have the technology yet.

In adept healers, the SU(2) magneto-electric force operates at a much greater magnitude than in ordinary people. How much greater? In 1992, Tiller teamed up with fellow scientist Elmer Green at The University of Kansas to assess the unique qualities and attributes of master healers. What they found was that whenever a healer "intended" a healing, electrodes across the healer's body measured a huge change in potential. In their paper "Towards Explaining Anomalously Large Body Voltage Surges on Exceptional Subjects Part I: The Electrostatic Approximation," Tiller and Green report the master healer's readings, showing dips of approximately 30–300 volts before returning to a baseline within 0.5–10 seconds.[232] This astoundingly large body voltage pulse is about 100,000 times the norm. In contrast, ordinary people show a baseline reading of 10–15 millivolts (mV) with 1 mV ripples.

Tiller's calculations with standard mathematics showed that these potentials appear to be magnetoelectric; they behave as magnetic potentials, which induce electric currents that then can be measured. Furthermore, he deduced that the measurements from point locations on the healer's body show flow along invisible lines within the body that correspond to known acupuncture meridian channels.

The acupuncture system potential can also be yours for the taking.[233] Become like a healer. Instead of the small ripples, you can generate huge pulses that you can direct. This is your intention manifesting in your body's energetic systems. You don't require any gas discharge device test to prove it.

Just do it.

Go pump it.

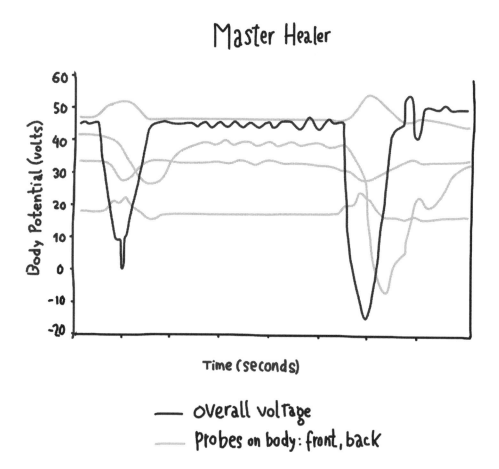

Master Healer

Overall voltage

Probes on body: front, back

[40]
"My research has led me to develop personal practices for subtle energy balancing and pumping."
The Eeman's Circuit

After serious injuries in a plane crash in World War I, British pilot Leon Ernest Eeman was deemed completely disabled beyond all hope of recovery and "permanently unfit for active duty." While hospitalized, he recalled Jesus's admonition: "Heal the sick by the laying on of hands."[234] Eeman reasoned that this healing energy was the subtle energy of the life force itself. He began to research methods to heal himself. Without medicines and surgeries, without any external sources of energy, and without yogic techniques, he came to discover the body's energy systems. Within two years after his release from the hospital, he had developed techniques, called "biocircuits" or "Eeman screens," that "restored him to better health than he had ever known." Eeman's book was republished in 1947 with the title *Cooperative Healing: The Curative Properties of Human Radiations.*[235]

Eeman showed that the body's energy systems could be connected by placing the left palm behind the head at the nape of the neck, the right palm over the sacrum, and the left ankle over the right. He called it the relaxation circuit. One Thursday meeting, Tiller introduced me to the Eeman's circuit. He gave me his handmade apparatus for completing the circuit, which I have kept and which I use every day. The process is simple and straightforward, even without the copper apparatus. The Eeman's circuit has saved me, literally, especially during the writing of this book. I travel frequently and my Eeman's device and my IHD go with me everywhere.

Tiller's apparatus makes completing the biocircuit easier on the hands because it has copper bars to hold on to; the copper bar for the left hand connects to a copper wire mat behind the head (base of the brain). The left side appears to be of one subtle energy polarity, while the base of the spine (sacral area) and the right hand appears to be of the opposite subtle energy polarity. Crossing my left ankle over the right, I soon sense pulsing, minute, current-like sensations in both hands. Most impressively, my scalp relaxes, and my mind is quiet like I am in meditation. Twenty minutes later, I rise feeling refreshed, like I've had a catnap. I have found it simple, safe, and effective. Every time.

In his white paper "Preventive Medicine/Self-Healing via One's Personal Biofield Pumping and Balancing," Tiller hypothesizes that the left hand draws energy from the head circuit, feeding it through the trunk of the body and out the right hand into the leg circuit.[236] In this way, the main information wave (subtle energy) circuits of the physical body are equalized, allowing the electric charge-based physical body to relax deeply. The copper wires serve as conductors of the subtle energy. It seems the body is characterized by a polarity, not unlike a magnet.[237]

In principle, you can learn to pump the subtle energy within your body using your hands. Lie on your left side with your head on a pillow and place your left hand on your neck at the base of the skull, your right palm on your tailbone. Cross your left ankle over your right. If you stay in this position for fifteen to twenty minutes, your body will have a relaxation response.

Time to rest on my Eeman's circuit.

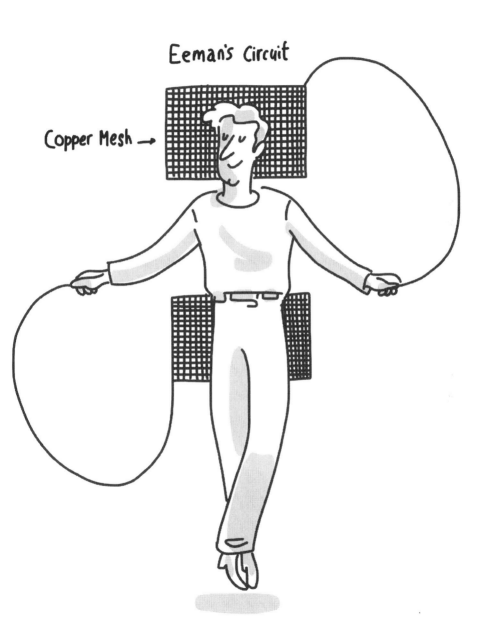

[41]
"Healing spaces can be created where people feel safe and well."
Healing Spaces and Negentropy at Your Doctor's Office

Imagine a world where your doctor's business card will state: "Our clinic is a conditioned space." Or where there are healing spaces specifically designed for ailments. Just go in and soak it up! It is a custom inventor's garage effect for health. Once you've gone in and soaked up excess energy, the clinic space recharges itself with an IHD onsite, by receiving a broadcast, or simply from the physicians and staff pumping it up with their intentions and healing activities.

Tiller's physics measures how conditioned a space is by calculating the excess free energy ΔG of the hydrogen ion (ΔG^*_{H+}). The water's pH is like an indicator or meter of how high above U(1) gauge, normal reality, a space is and its excess free thermodynamic energy.[238] For brevity, I will call it ΔG^*_{pH}. Energy flows spontaneously along the gradient from the higher ΔG^*_{pH} in a room space, to the lower ΔG^*_{pH} of a physical body's material atom/molecular "stuff," supplying energy for healing work.

A clinic can be tested to determine the strength and effectiveness of its space for healing work by measurement of ΔG^*_{pH}. This kind of real-world experiment was done in 2005 for a private start-up complementary and integrative medicine (CIM) clinic in Scottsdale, Arizona, as reported in Tiller's paper "Towards General Experimentation and Discovery in 'Conditioned' Laboratory and CAM [Complementary and Alternative Medicine] Spaces, Part V: Data on Ten Different Sites Using a Robust New Type of Subtle Energy Detector."[239]

A pH meter was used to continuously monitor one specific treatment room within the CIM clinic. Shifts in measurements of free hydrogen ions (H+) by the ΔG^*_{pH} throughout the day in real-time were collected as clients checked in and received their treatment. The pH meter continually recorded the ΔG^*_{pH} data during the night when no one was present and during weekends when the clinic was closed. Data was evaluated weekly.

The data pattern of ΔG^*_{pH} is compelling. To help you grasp the basic aspects, let's say we begin a regular clinic week on a Monday. The pH meter in the treatment room registers a steady level of ΔG^*_{pH}. The doors open on Monday and five clients check in. They each receive a treatment in the room. The ΔG^*_{pH} monitor is collecting data all the while. With each successive client, the pH meter shows a distinct dip in meV, indicating a decrease in free energy of the room. At the end of Monday, there are five dips, shaped by each person's treatment in the room. The clinic closes for the night, and the ΔG^*_{pH} graph shows an increase in meV free energy close to but not completely at the baseline.

The clinic reopens on Tuesday. Eight clients are booked on this day. As a client is treated, the excess free energy dips, usually by about 8–10 meV, with a distinct pattern. The clinic closes for the day and once again the data show a steady increase in ΔG^*_{pH} to a slightly lower level than the previous night. On Wednesday, the doors reopen, new clients check in, and the pattern repeats. The greater the number of clients, the greater the reduction or depletion of ΔG^*_{pH}. It takes about two days without any clients for the room's free energy, as measured by the ΔG^*_{pH}, to fully replenish the baseline levels to pre-treatment levels, ready for another week. Tiller gathered data for six weeks total.

With his protocol and data, Tiller demonstrated a method to quantify space conditioning and get new information about the "quality" of space, whether in a medical clinic, a physics laboratory, a hospital space, or in your garage, and that these measurements can be generalized into thermodynamic parameters. Measuring this quality may show whether a space is a good healing environment by providing a number, a quantity, of free energy.

In experimental work at Florida Atlantic University (FAU), as outlined in their paper "Altering the Acid/Alkaline Base of Water Via the Use of an Intention-Host Device," Grazyna Pajunen and Tiller monitored the water pH and ΔG^*_{pH} of a space in the university.[240] They reported that the pH rise lost momentum during examination time university-wide and by the time of the holiday season in December 2006, another period of stress, the pH had flattened and even trended downward. At the end of the first week in January 2007, one FAU researcher performed reiki, an intention-initiated energetic healing modality, for an extended period of time on a client. This healing session took place in the suite adjoining the experiment room. Subsequently, the pH values were observed to rise directly in a straight linear course.

All healing practices share a common premise, whether a practitioner is an MD from Yale or a shaman from Tibet: Your doctor is always pumping his space, even though he may not consciously know it. He is also supplying healing information by his spoken words and medical instructions that strengthens or corrects the complex processes already at work in our bodies.

Tiller explains: "Any interaction or relationship in the doctor's office involves information exchange, and any new information leads to a lowering of the entropy and thereby increases available excess energy. This is negentropy. This is not just behavioral expectation changes on part of the patient but real effects in terms of information exchange."

In the abstract of Tiller's paper, a motivation for the subtle energy detector is spelled out: This new understanding from this general body of work is important to all integrative medicine practitioners because it carries them beyond chemical medicine and even electromagnetic medicine in their practices. It allows them to seriously enter the domain of Information Medicine®. It allows them to utilize specifically imprinted IHDs for both research and treatment purposes. In the future, monitoring their clinic space will allow them to gain a quantitative measure of the "sacredness" of that space as a healing space. The term "sacred" is not precise here, but it is appropriate and meaningful.[241]

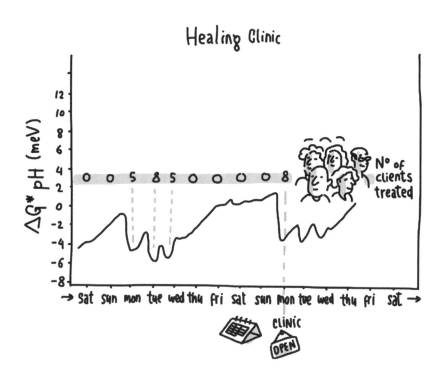

[42]
"Information Medicine is the way of the future."
Mama, I Love You

In the realm of psychoenergetics, Tiller has been particularly interested in distance healing. In his view: "It views the mind as unbounded and unconfined to points in space and time, so that this category of healing events may bridge persons who are widely separated from each other. This category of medicine goes well beyond today's view of physics so that mind, not matter, is ultimately considered as being primary."

Tiller's overall strategy is to use a specifically imprinted IHD to broadcast information to a group of individuals. One of the first broadcast programs was to care for the difficult and perplexing childhood disorder of autism. He calls the broadcast "Information Medicine."

The Centers for Disease Control and Prevention in the US estimate the prevalence of autism at one in fifty-nine children.[242] Millions have been spent on biomedical research for answers to the many types of autism. *The Diagnostic and Statistical Manual of Mental Disorders* lists the symptoms of autism as developmental delay, speech impediment, reduced social interaction, repetitive behavior; a list of attributes both abnormal and, often, difficult. There is a great deal of discussion nowadays about the correct medical treatment for these children. It is a sometimes heated and often misguided debate. In short, is something "broken" in a child with autism? Is there a chemical breakdown of some sort we can fix with a pharmaceutical drug? I think it's indicative of the way medicine sees the kids we label "disabled."

The reality of Information Medicine is grounded in the intention data and it provides an exciting possibility for autistic children. The intention research is translated from the laboratory bench to the bedside in order to tackle the real-world issue. It's the same pieces, be it water pH, a biological enzyme, or the fruit fly. Subtle energy characteristics underpin Information Medicine. Tiller went for the moonshot.

Tiller partnered with Suzy Miller, a speech and language pathologist certified by the American Speech and Hearing Association and author of the book *Awesomism!*[243] Miller is an expert in autism spectrum disorders. With Miller's expertise, he concentrated on crucial aspects that informed his intention statement creation with an emphasis on domains listed in the Autism Treatment Evaluation Checklist (ATEC): communication skills, sociability, cognitive awareness, and physical state.[244]

Tiller created this intention statement:[245]

"The special tuning characteristic for this IHD is to strongly increase the coupling between the D-space and R-space substances in each child's bedroom as well as in their own physical and subtle bodies so as to:

"Significantly reduce any impedance or information mismatch between their D-space and R-space bodies in their personality self,

"Significantly increase their desire that coherent connections develop between their various bodies for easy information exchanges between them, and

"Allow the radiation of divine love, divine joy, divine will, divine forgiveness, divine light, and divine wisdom to penetrate every nook and cranny of their being so as to significantly reduce all unnecessary stress precursors in their life, allowing them to manifest optimum health and functioning in physical, emotional, mental, and spiritual levels in their daily life, consistent with their soul's purpose for this particular lifetime's experience!"

Tiller created information in the old language of the heart. He did not specify an increase in the children's speech because, as Miller explained, "It was the last thing we expected to improve."

Another crucial piece in the design of this Information Medicine program was that Tiller made a controversial but definitive decision: "There will not be any controls. When we do something from the heart, it doesn't make sense to have controls."

The imprinting comes next. Along with Walter Dibble, Tiller imprinting team member Greg Fandel, and Tiller's wife, Jean, Tiller imprinted a device with the above intention for autistic children. The IHD was protected, wrapped in aluminum foil, and stored in a Faraday cage. Meanwhile, Miller reached out to families with autistic children located all around America and the globe, some as far away as Finland and Australia. Thirty-nine families signed a consent form to receive the intention broadcast over twelve months. The parents collected baseline and monthly data with the ATEC questionnaire about verbal skills, sociability, cognitive awareness, and physical state.

Tiller used a humble outfit; there was no medical center. Instead, the IHD was located in a small shed in Payson, among the pine trees. Tiller and Miller selected the day to switch on the IHD to begin the broadcast to the children, their names and addresses continually scrolling on a computer screen. Every sixty seconds, the next name popped up, and so on, around the clock. Like a laser beam, the intention information was broadcast to each child.

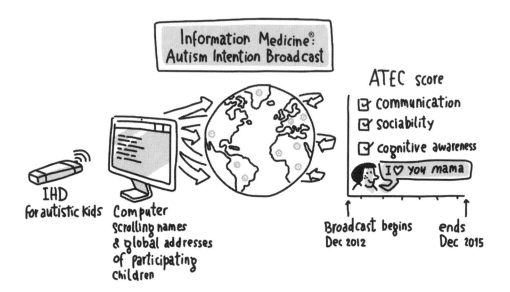

As noted in the white paper "The Globally Broadcast Autism Intention Experiment: Part 1, at the Four-Month Stage of a Twelve-Month Program," what happened next is the stuff of science fiction—except this is real science.[246] The first feedback arrived within twenty-four hours of switching on the IHD in Arizona. A mother from Australia called Miller: "My three-year-old! She said: 'I love you, Mama.'" The most this child had spoken in the past were nonsensical utterances and single words not necessarily appropriate for the situation. Moreover, the youngster spoke about twenty different words that day that were in perfect context. The mother exclaimed: "We all couldn't believe what we were hearing. Just amazing!"

Meanwhile, on the East Coast of the US, another child, a nine-year-old boy, was completely nonverbal as of the baseline on December 2, 2012, and functioning at a first-grade level (like a five-year-old). During the first few of months of the Information Medicine program, his mother indicated that he began to use facilitated communication, and he was able to explain things that she did not even know that he was aware of. His school test from October 2013 reported that he was satisfactorily functioning at a fifth-grade level (age ten to eleven in the US).[247]

Miller explained to me: "One of the predominate characteristics of autism is an inability to successfully use verbal language to communicate wants and needs. Science and education suggest that if an autistic child is nonverbal for neurological reasons, it is highly unlikely that they spontaneously recover their speech. It is also suggested that even with traditional therapy, the restoration of communication skills is typically a slow process. This is not, however, the case when children are worked with energetically."

During the Information Medicine broadcast, kids as old as fifteen who had never spoken began to form words. This is nothing short of amazing to an expert in the field. The kids improved, from 48 percent who could use four or more words to more than 60 percent in four months.[248] The children also began to show affection to their parents and siblings. In the abstract that Tiller coauthored with Miller, titled "Impact of Broadcast Intention on Autism Spectrum Behaviors," the differences in ATEC scores between the baseline and after Information Medicine are groundbreaking. The probability of the results is less than one in ten thousand, with a p-value less than 0.0001 for all subscales.[249] In the language of probability, these data mean less than one in ten thousand chance of being wrong. The benchmark for medical science is a p-value at or below 0.05, or a one-in-twenty chance. The information broadcast meets and exceeds that benchmark in all ATEC domains.[250]

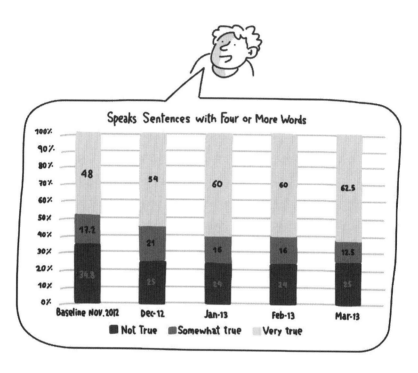

Remember, there is no direct sensory input from Tiller and these families, some of them thousands of miles away from Arizona. How does the intention information "know" which home to reach? How does information reach a precise home address in Australia? In Tiller's physics, the IHD initially "conditioned" his Payson shed space. This was strongly coupled (entangled) to transmit intention through R-space from Payson to each specific address being continuously scrolled on the laptop screen. In simpler terms, intention information reaches each home via R-space information entanglement. The families signed a consent form. They are part of the system. They are connected by field effects. It's like the Granny effect. The IHD was re-imprinted every three months to ensure that it remained metastable away from equilibrium.

There are still many questions. What happens to the space of the child's home itself? We don't know. Does a dose of intention of more than ten seconds mean greater change or faster change? In other words, is intention dose-dependent, to use the parlance of drug trials? Does more computer broadcast time to each child mean more "juice?" Amazingly, the children, through Miller, suggested that they did not need "more time" because they function outside of it. They function outside of time? Then it hit me. These children have psychoenergetic abilities like telepathy! These kids are not broken; they're simply streets ahead of us in their multidimensional consciousness. We cannot force them into our model of "normal." These children, even if nonverbal, have much to say and teach us.

When the full-length paper was submitted for publication, it was rejected. Reviewers raised objections about the lack of a control group of children and bias by confounding (self-selected families and parents). In my disappointment and feelings of futility on behalf of Tiller and Miller, I, together with the journal editors, had missed the point altogether. Bound up in the intricacies of the scientific method, of our academic demands and technology, we could not see that all the situation required was compassion. Not a solution to fix the children and their families, but a way to be kind and keep in touch, a way of reaching out to the suffering on the planet.

We can choose to hang back in the shadows and watch this whole experiment for a while, a physicist and young people in communion. In my view, the data is compelling and shows proof of concept of the feasibility of Information Medicine. However, the difficulties in publishing this sort of work are enormous. Suffice it to say that today's science remains firmly in its cause–effect paradigm. Ultimately, Tiller's choice not to have a control group shows his work comes from the heart, from something we call Love; a total surrender from a physicist who knew nothing of the families but knew of their struggle. He opened a door. Publishing and funding roadblocks do nothing to dampen Tiller's vision. He wants to help people and he does not experience burnout.

Tiller's response? "What they, the editors, think doesn't matter. When you perform God's work, do it from your heart. It doesn't make sense to have controls." The story is a familiar one from the days of Galileo:

> My dear Kepler, what would you say of the learned here, who, replete with the pertinacity of the asp, have steadfastly refused to cast a glance through the telescope? What shall we make of this? Shall we laugh or shall we cry?
>
> **–Letter from Galileo Galilei to Johannes Kepler** [251]

Yes, I am uneasy in my stance on Information Medicine, as early as it is in its history. But I am in favor of anything that introduces a little more empathy into the world. I would like to champion Information Medicine simply as one way to support people for whom we have few to no helpful answers. This is what I stand for. We in the scientific community have an opportunity to take this early work and propose steps to brings Information Medicine into a wider know-how.

There's a postscript. Tiller and Jean were, and continue to be, immensely touched by the letters and feedback from the children and their parents.

[43]
"Many people are deficient in self-acceptance."
Heart over Matter: Message in a Box

This ought to be the best of times for the human mind, but it is not so. It seems that life is full of promises unfulfilled. During the days and nights, as people go on with their daily lives, there seems to be a faint aura of disquiet in the air. This is making experts like Dr. Vivek Murthy, the nineteenth US Surgeon General, troubled. In an article in the *Harvard Business Review,* titled "Work and the Loneliness Epidemic: Reducing Isolation at Work Is Good for Business," Murthy spells it out: in America, loneliness is at epidemic levels. An estimated forty-four million Americans age forty-five and older experience chronic loneliness.[252] Many people put up apparent confidence as a mask for deep doubts about themselves and their ability to cope with the challenges and problems of living. Similarly, across the pond, in January 2018, British prime minister Theresa May appointed a new cabinet minister to tackle the problem of loneliness in the UK.[253]

A feeling of being alone in the world is, I feel, an issue of our individual and collective consciousness. I cannot begin to guess at all the causes of our cultural sadness, but I can think of one thing that is wrong with us: We do not know enough about ourselves. As long as we are befuddled by the mystery of ourselves and bewildered by the perplexity of our own minds, we cannot be said to be healthy animals in today's world.

In his book *Science and Human Transformation,* Tiller explains that the most profitable point on which to focus one's intention to engender sustainable human transformation is the heart, in the emotional sense. Furthermore, he writes that influxes in spiritual energy to a human being can, at best, be integrated and, at worst, become destabilizing if the heart is not developed enough to handle it. Therefore, the critical point for beneficially influencing human spiritual evolution is the heart.[254]

In partnership with psychologist Gabrielle Hilberg, PhD, MFT, Tiller turned to Information Medicine to broadcast self-compassion to people with loneliness. Self-compassion means being kind toward oneself in times of pain or failure, perceiving one's experiences as part of life's broader experience, and holding painful thoughts and feelings in balanced awareness. Thirty-nine people in Hilberg's practice signed a consent form to receive Information Medicine. The IHD, located in Payson, broadcast to the clients, most of whom live in San Francisco. By any outer measure, the participants, all with college degrees, are hugely successful. Yet many felt anxiety, a feeling of daily unease, and a lack of fulfillment.

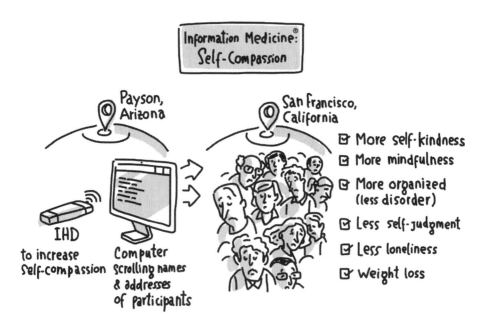

The Tiller intention broadcast included the following main parts:

1. An empowerment factor to diminish personal fear-fulness related to survival and self-image and to reduce self-grasping.

2. The intention to bring about incremental and sustainable gains in an individual's progress. The self-compassion broadcast provided a metaphorical staircase; each participant was presented with a new step on a staircase. They had to take the step up, and once they did, they remained on that step. Then the next step appeared, and so on from there. The details of the information statement are included in Appendix 3.

Participants' baseline scores on the primary measures: Neff Self-Compassion Scale (NEFF),[255] and Rosenberg Self-Criticism Test were collected.[256] To provide perspective, on the NEFF 1–5 scale, average overall self-compassion scores tend to be around 3.0. A score of 1–2.5 indicates low self-compassion, a score of 2.5–3.5 indicates moderate self-compassion, and 3.5–5.0 means high self-compassion. Over ten months, the IHD spread the "word without words" of the self-compassion intention around the clock, seven days a week. The average NEFF self-compassion score increased from 2.7 to 3.6, a difference that was significant, with a less than one in ten thousand probability of being by chance ($p < 0.0001$).[257]

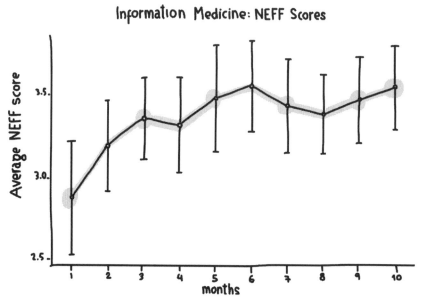

In the participants, all various data results met or exceeded the benchmark in medical research of a probability of improvement due to chance of one in twenty (also known as a p-value of 0.05). The eight metrics—self-kindness, self-judgment, sense of common humanity, sense of isolation, mindfulness, sense of equanimity, Rosenberg Self-Criticism Test score, and the Zung Depression Test score—all met or exceeded the probability benchmark at 0.05. These results speak powerfully of the effectiveness of Tiller's Information Medicine method.

Hilberg's own deduction is that, unlike other healing approaches, which focus on "fixing," Tiller's Information Medicine approach seems to ignite the self-healing potential within each participant. Remarkably, the intention broadcast "spilled" into their lives in more ways than treating loneliness. Testimonials to Hilberg included "greater tidiness," "more organized," "better food choices," "weight loss," "a sense of contentment," and a sense of "joyful living,"[258] even though all outer conditions remained unchanged.

Hilberg went on to share her observations that the Tiller approach is based on the belief that we can remember on a deep level who we really are. His healing information of unconditional Love could be thought of as activating consciousness at our soul level, thereby leading to a decrease in neurotic patterns held by the ego. Dr. David Hawkins calls this dropping of inimical behaviors "letting go."[259] Therefore, while we still have much to learn of the mechanism of Information Medicine effects, it appears fundamentally to catalyze shifts at multiple levels of being. One phase change and transformation leads to the next phase, on down to the thermodynamically new stable state.

Tiller's Information Medicine has offered something hard to find in medicine today: wisdom and unconditional Loving care. Much of medicine focuses on grievance and on disease, rather than guiding people toward a meaningful life. That a group of people would voluntarily submit themselves to this broadcast surely suggests that we crave meaning to ourselves and to others. Tiller's protocol provides it. It is also delivered 24/7, without any waiting room time, without risk of chemical side effects to body or nature. Tiller and Hilberg's intention is that the participants will "hear" something different. It touches us all.

This invisible force—Love—makes science uncomfortable. We can consider this force as impersonal as gravity. Love can be viewed as a force of nature, like entropy or molecular decay. Similarly, a call to Love can be conceptualized as personal or as impersonal, like the tides or the transiting of Venus. The point, for the thesis I'm seeking to put forward, is that there are forces within us and around us, and they are our allies in medicine and all endeavors.

[44]
"Information Medicine
is personalized medicine."
Where the Rubber Meets the Road:
Chemical, Energy, and Information Medicine

This part of the bridge serves an important function to connect concepts and closes a span in medicine of delivering personalized care, safely and potentially effectively, to achieve ideal outcomes for a specific client: a moonshot that won't cost the moon!

To highlight how the concepts of chemical (drug-based) medicine, energy medicine, and Information Medicine all fit together, I present a case report of my patient who suffers from a type of arthritis called "ankylosing spondylitis." In this disease, joints and the lower spine, particularly the sacral area, become inflamed and very painful, sometimes leading to disability. It often strikes males in the prime of life.

Mark lives in Minneapolis, Minnesota. He began to have trouble with arthritis in 1995, at the age of forty. By 2006, when I was his doctor, his health had deteriorated and he suffered almost constant pain in his elbows and knees, which he described as being an eight to nine out of ten on the pain scale, that is, severe. To search the cause of his pain, he made frequent visits to many specialists: rheumatology, neurology, pain management, sports medicine, rehabilitation, orthopedic surgery, and more. Diagnostic evaluations included numerous blood tests, X-rays, and magnetic resonance imaging (MRI) to delineate the anatomy of the tendons and joints.

He received the best of conventional medicine, with state-of-the-art biologics, a class of medications designed to target specific proteins that result in inflammation. Unfortunately, almost all treatments were unsuccessful in alleviating his pain. The biological medications had been discontinued in 2010 for lack of effect. By 2011, when I left this medical center, Mark was under the care of a team of physicians. Doctors wrote: "We don't know the etiology [cause] of his pain" and "we are running out of options."

The toll on Mark's quality of life was dramatic. He gave up his favorite winter sport of skiing and regular exercise and walking his dogs were out of the question. Out went the gym membership. His work as an executive required frequent traveling, which he suspended. He could not use his left arm because of searing elbow pain even with adjustments at his desk; his left arm withered as the muscles atrophied. He described his quality of life as miserable with fear and anxiety, and he was desperate for "something, anything, to be done."

In 2012, Mark contacted me. He was aware of my interest in energy medicine and with Tiller's experimental protocol. Mark was emphatic: "I want to try this approach [of information medicine]. Nothing else has helped." He understood that (1) information medicine does not have any clinical trial data (RCTs); (2) it isn't a medical therapy recognized by the Food and Drug Administration (FDA); and (3) he should not stop his medical care. Based on compassionate need, Tiller agreed to help him with the understanding that potential benefits outweighed potential risks and there was no guarantee of reducing pain. After signing a consent form to receive Information Medicine, Mark, with my assistance, outlined his wishes for optimal well-being: being pain-free and regaining his muscle strength. Tiller, Mark, and I reviewed the wish list until we all felt satisfied that it had the core aspects he wanted.

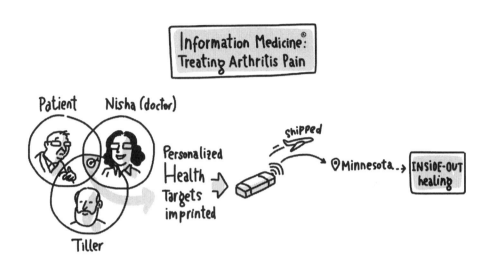

Tiller created an intention statement over several weeks. It drew on Mark's answers to questions like, "What is the best possible life that you can imagine?" Any obstacles Mark perceived were noted. All levels of well-being were addressed in the intention statement: physical, mental and emotional, and spiritual.

In summer of 2012, Tiller and his team imprinted a personalized IHD, which was protected and shipped to Mark's home in Minneapolis. He continued his conventional medical care as the Information Medicine program was underway, although his rheumatologist had discontinued the biologic and anti-inflammatory pharmaceuticals for more than two years in 2010 because of lack of effectiveness.[260]

Every three months, Tiller re-imprinted the personalized IHD to keep it "active" and metastable. Mark completed the Bath Ankylosing Spondylitis Disease Activity Index (BASDAI) questionnaire for ankylosing spondylitis which takes into account joint pain, morning stiffness, and areas of localized tenderness (inflammation of tendons and ligaments).[261] The BASDAI score ranges from 0 to 10. Scores of 4 or greater indicate active disease. At the start of the program, Mark's BASDAI score was 8, indicating severe and active ankylosing spondylitis.

Using Tiller's terminology, Mark's treatment regimen consisted of:

☐ Chemical, conventional medicine consisting of pharmaceuticals to impact atoms/molecules (D-space), partial list:

  » Ceased use two years prior to starting Information Medicine:
  - sulfasalazine tablets to control the immune-mediated joint and tendon inflammation
  - biologic medication: adalimumab (Humira®) injections & etanercept (Enbrel®) injections
  - gabapentin (Neurontin®) to ease nerve pain

  » Continued to use:
  - Acetaminophen (Tylenol®) for pain
  - Ibuprofen (Advil®) for anti-inflammation
  - topical compounded anesthetic cream with amitriptyline, ketamine, and clonidine
  - injections of steroids and anesthetic into affected joints
  - surgical removal of a small (6 mm) benign lymph node at the left elbow thought to cause pain
  - a rigorous anti-inflammatory diet combined with supplements such as turmeric, essential fatty acids (omega-3 oils), and ashwagandha for resiliency

☐ Energy medicine (D-space and R-space): External hands-on qigong healing from a master healer, often with dramatic but short-lived (usually 24 to 48 hour) reduction in pain.

☐ Information Medicine (R-space): Personalized IHD

The IHD delivered a customized information broadcast into Mark's bedroom. Within the first month or two, he began to have what I call "inside-out" healing. His emotions lifted and he was feeling more optimistic. However, the joint and tendon pain, his physical body, lagged behind the inner processes. It took about thirty-six months until the physical pain improved suddenly. As Mark reported to me in June 2018: "For no apparent reason, my pain has disappeared." For the first time since the start of his arthritis in 1995, he could tolerate a consistent rehabilitation program to rebuild muscle tissue. His BAS-DAI score at the time of this writing decreased on a ten-point scale from 8 to 3.5, which indicates remission. He remains off of biologic medicines.

I feel compelled to register at least a note of *Homo dubitat*. Sudden remissions and miraculous cures are notoriously difficult to assess. Was this just coincidence? Maybe it was a hiatus, an upswing. Chronic illnesses can go up and down. However, his long history of poor outcomes over the twelve years I have known him, and the absence of significant improvement from powerful biologic medications for several years makes it unlikely it was an "upswing." From my clinical experience as a rheumatologist, there is currently no data to support spontaneous remission in ankylosing spondylitis.

Why did the Information Medicine program take long to show the desired pain reduction? Tiller felt that what Mark was going through was not entirely at the physical level. Indeed, if it were, then the conventional treatment for joint and tendonitis inflammation would have worked. Nor was the issue just at the acupuncture meridian system because, again, the relief Mark experienced after external qigong from a master healer would have been sustained.

According to Tiller, Mark's symptoms were beyond both the physical body and the acupuncture system. He believes the healing in-formation from the IHD broadcast improved Mark's being at deep levels, cascading down from the R-space of his acupuncture system to the gross body level. Even during the so-called "dry periods" where nothing appeared to change, there was likely improvement continu-ally occurring in all levels of Mark's being.

In terms of thermodynamics, we can think of the physical body like the topography of space. In the beginning, a person has a certain topography, an initial starting phase. First, a thermodynamic free en-ergy driving force for a change builds up in the topography of mag-netic vector phase change. Next, a partially deconstructed original structure is followed by a rearrangement of the primary structural elements into a new configuration amenable to lowering the exist-ing thermodynamic free energy driving force. The transforming pro-cesses repeat until all the excess thermodynamic free energy driving force (created by the IHD) has been used up.

Thus, one observes something of a successive sequence of phase changes in geological structure slowly over time until $\Delta G=0$ and the thermodynamically stable stage, optimal health, is formed. Of course, this may take thousands to millions of years to occur. And sometimes the chain of reactions does not even reach optimal because the kinet-ics of structural change are too slow.[262]

Tiller feels that another reason for the extended time to physical response could be that intention moves slowly because, in some sit-uations, that is the right way to do things. All things unfold in God's time and for the highest good. Tiller takes action and surrenders out-comes or time. I think with the personalized broadcast, Mark's un-conscious was given a brand new highly complex set of instructions, and he had an inside-out process that took the time necessary for a new physical body to emerge.

Tiller was not manipulating anything (and he has never personally met Mark), but it is a reminder that in our biological system, almost anything can happen. Mark feels convinced that, all things being equal, and without any of the intense pharmaceutical prescription drugs for more than six years, that the IHD had a positive impact on his health without side effects or astronomical costs. There are many people like Mark who, despite the tremendous progress in immunology and new medicines to treat arthritis, have little or no response to modern therapeutics.

In summary, an overall thermodynamic principle can be bridged and constructed: There are increasing levels of thermodynamic free energy from chemical to energy medicine, higher still to Information Medicine (IHD), and finally the highest source of ΔG, which is Spirit. From Spirit, there is a cascade of healing energy down through all the levels, nourishing the meridians and the physical body. To advance and enhance modern healthcare, healing on all levels is important.

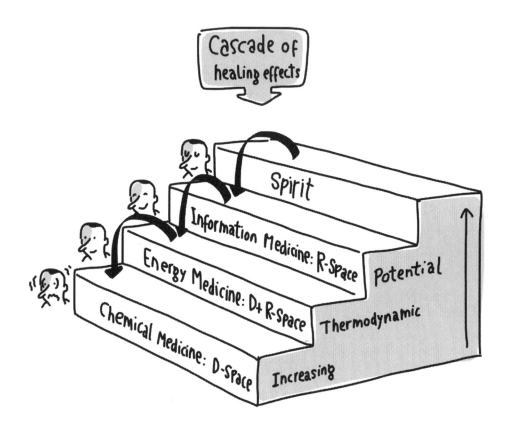

[45]
"Consciousness beats lifestyle."
Your Intention Matters to Your Health and Well-Being

Humans are constantly retooling and rebuilding themselves for a healthy life. Lifestyle factors like exercise, organic foods, and relationships contribute to a healthy life. Meditation and mindfulness have become household words. Rarely, however, is the level of consciousness factored in.

If we use the Hawkins Map of Consciousness, it is estimated that on average, a human being's level of consciousness increases five points (on a scale of 0 to 1,000) in a lifetime.[263] This consciousness scale is logarithmic with a base of ten. This means a one-point increase is equivalent to ten times the power of the number below it. An increase of five points signifies a gain of 10^5, one hundred thousand times the power. As one degree increase in temperature can turn water to steam, a very different phenomenon from liquid, a five-point increase in consciousness represents a significant shift in inner perception.

There is more to the story of the information broadcast for the autistic children. Experienced kinesiologists in Edmonton, Canada, who were blinded to the group and did not know about the intention broadcast, monitored the consciousness level of the children and their parents. "Blind" is a term used in clinical trials describing testers who, to ensure objectivity, do have not have information about test subjects that can cause data bias. The two-person team doing the muscle testing followed the steps in Appendix 2 and tested statements specifically, "information" of the increase in points in the levels of consciousness.

The autistic children and their parents experienced a ten-point increase in their consciousness level in the first twelve months of the Information Medicine broadcast. It's *yowza* all over again. Ten points on the consciousness scale means a 10^{10} or *10 billion times* increase in power! The body looks the same, wearing the same clothes. But the kids are different. The mothers are different, the fathers are different.

This jump in consciousness means the development of the children and their parents was expedited. Their load in this lifetime was lightened and their evolution quickened. This is healing from the inside-out, and more than that, it is a metamorphosis. Tiller's information program was like a spiritual balm and first aid for the families. The recipients' informational infrastructure was forever altered.

Tiller says: "Generally, what happens if we create new information in ourselves, build it into ourselves, and if we meditate, [is that] we go deep into the silence, and that's called inner-work. We become more and more coherent. Then we see the consequence of being more coherent regarding our energy capacity, which can go up by orders of magnitude." And who doesn't want more energy!

Consciousness is not a thing, but a process of personal growth and registering new experiences. As we value experiences above things, we get more conscious and more open to more profound and more complex experiences. We all know the immense progress in machine learning. What remains to be seen is the progress of human consciousness: How fast and deep will it go?

What does this mean for you and me? The level of consciousness is the most crucial aspect in health. I'd wager it will improve relationships, improve our self-esteem, lift us up to really live, all without drugs. Our level of consciousness is that part of us that is unsullied. It is waterproof, fireproof, age proof, bulletproof.

If the mystics say that our primary purpose in life is growing in consciousness, then the intention broadcast marks very significant progress in science and medicine. It is revolutionary.

As conscious humans, we have a responsibility. We cannot remain *Homo dubitat* for much longer. We must act and overthrow the programming of our cellphones, unplug from the TV. We are being called to become alert, awake, in charge.

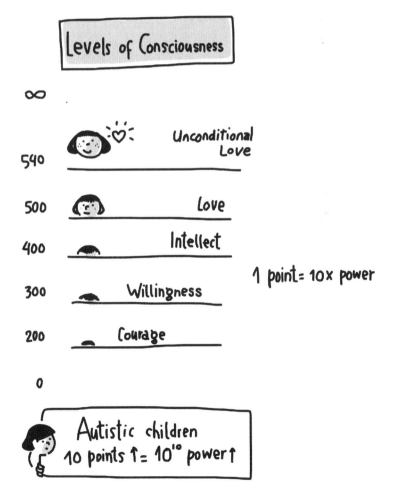

Now, from the standpoint of a new perspective, the gap again intervened in the known world and a new world that is relevant to you and me. I want to go to the other side. The world takes on an obscurity. A new problem presents itself in the form: "How may these pillars be joined, this time from the other side?

—Franklin Merrell-Wolff

in *Pathways through to Space: An Experiential Journal* [264]

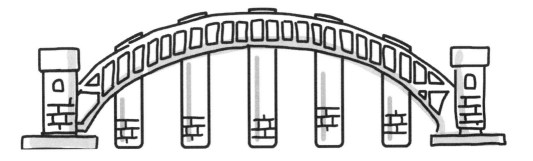

BRIDGE PILLAR 7:
Of Thermodynamics, Love, and Becoming *Homo spiritus*

Geniuses are the luckiest of mortals because what they must
do is the same as that as what they most want to do and,
even if their genius is unrecognized in their lifetime, the essential
earthly reward is always theirs, the certainty that their work is good
and will stand the test of time. One suspects that the geniuses
will be least in the Kingdom of Heaven—if, indeed,
they ever make it; they have had their reward.

—W.H. AUDEN, from the opening page of *A Mind at Play: How Claude Shannon Invented the Information Age* by Jimmy Soni and Rob Goodman[265]

Science is a way to self-knowledge.
—WILLIAM A. TILLER[266]

[46]
"It is not a traditional force that radiates from the relics of the historical Buddha."
Consciousness without a Brain: The Buddha Relics

Aristotle had a word for it: metaphysics. Literally, beyond physics. As a philosophical science, metaphysics takes its name from the idea that it goes beyond "hard" science into the realm of transcendental concepts such as the nature of existence, as well as moral and intellectual speculation, where no empirical proof is possible. For example, how can things exist and also undergo change? Aristotle believed that in every change there is something that persists through the change.

When I started my Thursday meetings with Tiller, I was sure the most important questions in life couldn't be answered by pure scientific reason. Tiller defended his belief in both: a higher order, the Unseen and "mythos," and the world of logic and the intellect which he calls "logos." From the intellectual domain of logos, we cross the bridge span to the Spirit side. The final pillar returns us to ourselves and asks how to think about our existence and spirituality in the light of the extraordinary world described by the target experiments.

Spirit has come to us in the form of the historical Buddha's relics. The relics, known as *ringsel* in Tibetan, resemble small crystal-like pearls. They appear during the cremation of some Buddha Masters, embodying all the divine attributes of the master: a crystallized manifestation of unconditional Love, compassion, and wisdom.

The relics of Shakyamuni Buddha, who died in the fifth century BC, have survived for more than 2,500 years. After being saved in Tibet and various monasteries in Asia, the precious relics were brought from Tibet with His Holiness the Fourteenth Dalai Lama during his escape to India in 1959. Extraordinarily, in 2001, these relics were exhibited over a fourteen-year public tour, visiting all five continents, with an estimated two million viewers. My personal experience of viewing the precious relics in Gyuto Wheel of Dharma Monastery in Minneapolis was thus:[267]

> Upon entering the monastery, I immediately felt an intense state of awareness or presence. It was as though the Buddha himself was present. The state was nonverbal, vast, and profound; it was exquisitely gentle and yet like a rock. There was a silence and a state of peace that seemed limitless. For me, the essence of time ceased to exist. My mind became quieter, for in place of the usual internal conversation was wonder, and curiosity had given way to amazement. I felt a tangible radiation of exquisite energy flowing from the relics to my heart center. It was highly private and personal, and yet conveyed an immense sense of oneness or unity with everyone and everything. It had no counterpart in ordinary experience.

Astoundingly there was nobody, "no-body," present, no flesh, bone, or brain in front of me. Yet the Buddha, by way of his relics, interacted with me, loved me, talked with me, gave me intuitions about questions I was holding in my mind, in an all-pervading field of unconditional Lovingness radiating, broadcasting, from his relics in the stupas. Buddha's relics forced me to question all my notions and answers about the brain being the seat of consciousness.[268]

When I (sort of) recovered, my brother Raj and I made the firm intention to invite the relics of the Buddha Masters to our family home. We were granted permission, and the Maitreya Project relics were exhibited for three days at our home in Southern California. The moment the Buddha's relics entered our home, the ordinary living room swiftly, within a few seconds, felt like the interior space of a high cathedral, like Westminster Abbey!

Over the three days, an estimated 3,500 visitors came through our home to view the sacred relics: neighbors, friends, pets, children, and people from all walks of life. Many visitors reported feelings of emotional, physical, and mental "lifting," as though a heavy burden had been relieved. Others reported being "washed" deeply from the "inside out" to a peaceful state. A few minutes in the presence of the sacred relics and people emerged, faces transformed. Words fail to adequately describe the exceptional shifts in visitors.

Here is an example of objects—sacred relics—that are conscious and intelligent, giving a vital clue that consciousness can exist without a body or brain. Here is the vital clue to a higher level of nature existing over vast periods of clock time. Usual methodologies, like MRI imaging, cannot answer fundamental questions about the nature of the Buddha's relics. The general lack of information about relics in scientific literature and the nature of my inquiry made it necessary for me to draw heavily on Tiller's subtle energy research and the consistency of the reports I find there. Note the straightforward parallels between the Buddha's relics and Tiller's IHD:

Buddha's Relics	Tiller's Intention Host Device (IHD)
Relic "pearl-like object" device	Simple circuitry-electric device
Protected in small stupas and wrapped in ceremonial Tibetan scarves	Wrapped and protected in aluminum foil
Transported to displays in different cities for public "lifting"	Transported to labs in different cities for experiments
Metastable for more than 2,600 years	Metastable for more than six months
Conditions space within a few seconds	Conditions space within a few weeks or months

The first question is, what kind of radiation is emitted from the Buddha's relics? If we stop for a moment and consider that thousands of people report experiences of healing and emotional transformation, whatever that radiation might be, it is not a conventional force like electromagnetism. Maxwell's equations do not describe these subtle energies. Second, qualitatively, I can unequivocally state that the relics are a repository of the Buddha's intention of unconditional Loving-kindness. The broadcast from the relics is like being hugged by your grandmother, totally, tightly, a bosom hug. An unconditional, heart-to-heart hug. The Buddha left behind profound gifts of loving-kindness for the benefit of all sentient beings. Once you've had a taste of Loving-kindness, it feels like coming home. This is our true existence and reality.

We enter an entirely new territory. We are dealing here with something that is "holy" in the strict sense of that word, which was first used to describe that which was "healthy and intact." It seems to me a relic from generations past is an object dedicated to a given end that seeks completion in its own special way, restless until it reaches equilibrium. It is different than Tiller's IHD, the electrical equivalent, but the latter, too, becomes something incomplete unless it has achieved its particular end given to it by man, and restless until it reaches equilibrium.[269]

The question of what the relics are made of is unimportant. What matters is that we share a common sensitivity and are able to respond in some way to a set of stimuli that give certain objects a necessary, special, and magical quality.

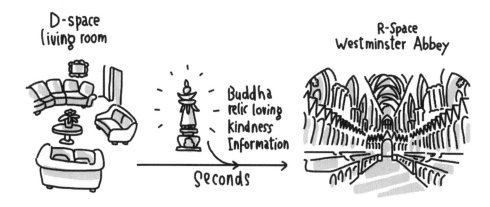

[47]
"Thermodynamics of loving-kindness can be measured."
Love That Burns

Experientially, the Buddha relics rapidly condition or "lift" space where they are exhibited. When the Maitreya tour exhibited at our home, I saw an opportunity to "capture" the Loving-kindness essence and activate Tiller's UEDs. During those three days, several of Tiller's UEDs were placed underneath the table on which the Buddha Masters' relics were kept. I did not write a statement for the imprinting process. Rather, I intuited that placing the UEDs demonstrated my intention tangibly. In this way, the subtle energy information of Buddha's Loving-kindness "activated" to convert the UEDs to IHDs, which I designated as "ReIHD" for "Relic-IHD." All ReIHDs were wrapped individually with aluminum foil and stored safely. I proposed to Tiller that we could test my hypothesis that Buddha's relics condition an ordinary D-space to R-space by utilizing one of the ReIHDs and measuring the change in water pH (ΔG^*_{pH}).

Tiller proceeded with the experiment with one of the ReIHDs. First, he gathered the background data of the unconditioned test space for two weeks: ultra-pure water pH and temperature and the room air temperature, with continual digital data recording. Then Tiller positioned the ReIHD a few inches from the water vessel setup. One day went by. Nothing happened, and the pH remained steady at equilibrium per thermodynamic calculations for D-space.[270] One day stretched into one week, then two weeks. Still no water pH shift materialized. Zilch. Nothing.

My brother and I had already witnessed the Buddha relics "lift" the space in our home in a few seconds. Yet, here we were in week two.

I was aghast.

I pondered the apparent "failure" of our protocol before Tiller arrived for our Thursday meeting. Then, unexpectedly, the answer hit me like a thunderbolt, like Buddha himself was pointing the way! Even today, I am absolutely astounded with the implications.

The relics were conditioning the space to such a high level that Tiller's experimental setup, designed for SU(2) space, was *unable* to register the much higher-order gauge symmetries. The Buddha's relics are more powerful, and the ReIHD could reasonably be expected to condition space to a higher-gauge symmetry than SU(2). Our protocol was inadequate. We didn't have *adaequatio*.

What could we do now?

Jean Tiller, about the same time, suggested a modification. She said to Tiller: "You have to ask the ReIHD specifically what you want. Just plugging in [the ReIHD] is insufficient. You have to write an intention inviting the intelligence of the ReIHD to be measurable."

Tiller promptly got to work. The only logical approach was to treat the ReIHD like a living thing. He wrote: "We respectfully request that the excess thermodynamic free energy aspect of this Loving-kindness essence be made manifest in this space so that we can experimentally measure its thermodynamic magnitude via the active pH sensors present in this space."

What happened next is the stuff of miracles and science fiction rolled into one. The water pH meter took off. Immediately. We watched the data come in, enthralled. The pH units adding up, and the experiment—ReIHD and water pH meter—seemed to have an intelligence, almost seeming to answer us from beyond clock-time. It was magnificent and something more, something that made this experiment almost unreal. The ΔpH climbed one unit, then two units in two weeks, and was going strong, the water pH slope steep, with little deviation.[271]

It was unambiguous. *We had been answered in such grace that it only served to emphasize our connection to God beyond all time, and the perfection of Tiller's call and personal prayerful petition.*

All this time later—seven years, it is hard to believe this result happened. We checked with each other and all had felt the same excitement. Tiller put it best. Shaking his head, he said wonderingly: "I didn't know . . ." My reaction: *Yowza!* The change in water ΔpH with the ReIHD was an increase of 2.5 units, representing 60 meV. In thermal terms, a room temperature of 700 °C would be required for such a vigorous ΔpH. The room would literally burn up!

What was going on here?

Tiller said: "It could be only one thing, one term of the second law. The most profound change was informational, the reduction in entropy by the Loving-kindness information." As we know, acquiring new information represents a decrease in entropy and an increase in free energy. The change in water pH yielded a number over the course of two weeks for the increase in excess free energy. This, my friends, is thermodynamics of unconditional Loving-kindness information. The excess energy is from coherence in the physical vacuum, a lessening of entropy, or in other words, negentropy.

An apparently failed protocol led to an unbelievable, more fantastic moment. At its heart is a culmination of ideas all centered on the notion that seeming inanimate objects, like ReIHDs, that are inorganic in every other respect seem to satisfy the usual requirements of life, of consciousness, and, yes, of intelligence.

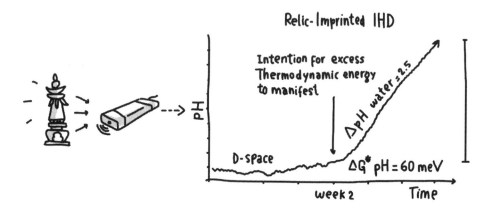

[48]
"The Buddha relics show us the answer to mankind's age-old question: Does consciousness survive physical death?"
A Primal Question Answered

As a doctor, I am trained to identify the criteria of life and distinguish the living from the dead by restricting my attention to a body's physical systems. Currently, medicine would state that when a person dies, life ends because core chemical processes that underlie existence—the heartbeat, breath, and brain activity—are disrupted and cease. Medical science rarely delves into the possibility that consciousness may survive after physical death. By and large, these questions have been relegated to the metaphysical domain and are beyond my concern as a physician. For something like consciousness to be present in an inanimate object (like a relic) that has been around for more than 2,500 years and is ostensibly "alive" seems outrageous. But it is no longer possible to be so circumscribed, for "things," even the inorganic and undeniably inanimate, sometimes behave as though they were alive, even sentient. Life, it seems to me, is not so easily defined exclusively by the processes of a physical body.

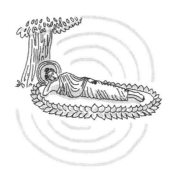

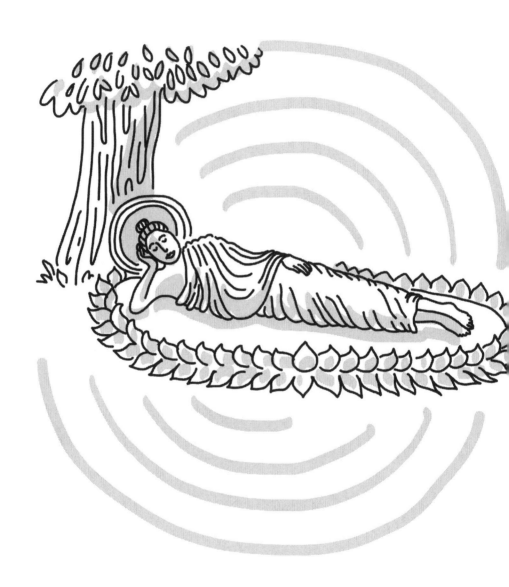

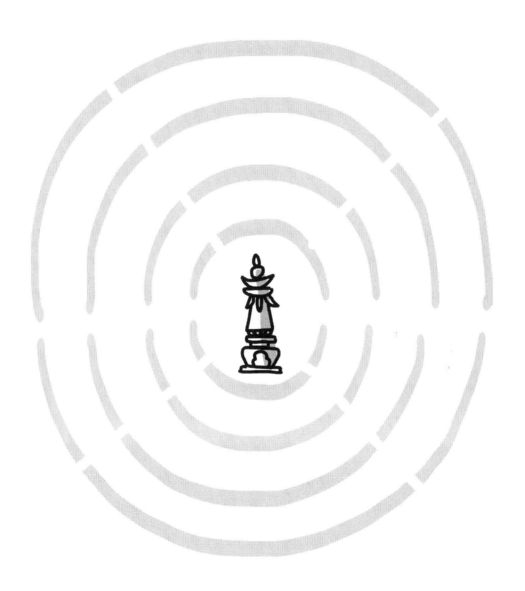

[49]
"Nothing is causing anything."
Potentiality Becomes Actuality

This causes that. This is a fundamental assumption of science. It is a fundamental assumption you and I have about the universe. You throw a ball and it sails across your yard. You think you "caused" the ball to move against gravity to a location. Then, by playing fetch, your dog causes the ball to come back to you.

Or take a seed that you plant: You water it, and allow it plenty of sunshine, and the potential in the seed is actualized to a marigold. You cannot force the seed to sprout; you cannot shout at it to grow; you cannot make the seed do anything. You simply create the conditions by planting it in the optimal setting and the marvelous hidden unmanifest potential in the seed is actualized. Your actions of planting a seed seem to reduce causality to an expression of human agency. Yet, millions of variables interact for your marigold seed to actualize its magnificence, factors beyond the discernable and explicit forms, to the formless and infinite.

The idea of a "this causing that" is built so deeply into our pattern of thinking that we can't just step outside of it and consider a universe without it. The question of why the universe appears causal is very difficult to discuss, not to mention answer satisfactorily. But this is a crucial brick in the bridge. This idea that nothing is causing anything gets us to the other side of the bridge faster.

Tiller didn't force the water pH to change with chemicals, nor did he force the *Drosophila* fruit fly larvae to mature faster. Instead, he created the conditions, the field, that allowed the potentiality of the larvae to mature faster. Nothing was forced. Tiller didn't cause any-thing. All phenomena of the target experiments emerged as a conse-quence of their potentiality, if conditions were favorable.

The notion of favorable conditions brings us back to probabilities. In theory, the starting point of a device being imprinted with infor-mation, which in turn could be used to change something in physical reality, had very long odds. But, of course, it was not a random pro-cess. Tiller's skill and intent twisted the odds, favoring the chosen lab space, giving one spot a very special significance and making it different from any other space. That R-space field, acting as an in-formational blueprint, shaped the material stuff contained in it, the atoms and molecules, into a nonequilibrium state, an assembly of an altogether different complexity in line with Tiller's directive. And what we saw was the odds of the anomalous, of the improbable, being nudged to a less improbable event.

In thermodynamic terms, Tiller has presented the case for the hy-pothesis that a steady flow of intention and subtle energy from the bountiful source of the heart, by way of the device, is mathemati-cally destined to increase the chances of a different ordered state. It was thermodynamically inevitable that it must rearrange matter away from probability, against entropy, "lifting" it, so to speak, into a changing rearrangement and molecular ornamentation. The outcome could have descended to disarray, but it was held taut against prob-ability by the laser-like information and surge of subtle energy from the IHD.

For the correct and consistent description of Tiller's refined expe-rience, we need to change the conceptual link between the microscop-ic and macroscopic worlds. We do not normally encounter intention effects in a spacetime-only world because of statistical considerations of the Boltzmann's constant, *k,* which is a tiny number. Recall that Boltzmann's constant connects the microscopic and the macroscopic worlds. In D-space, *k* is 1.38 x 10^{-23} joules/Kelvin. Tiller postulates that the analog of *k,* in R-space, is smaller by a factor of 10^6 (one million). This means entropy, *S,* decreases. The probability of fruit fly larvae maturing faster is increased.

A scientific constant is just that: constant and unchanging. Or is it? Physicists have speculated that constants, such as the gravity constant, change in small ways that we are unable to detect. It is not unreasonable to think that the Boltzmann constant is different in R-space. In 2019, the *Bureau international des poids et mesures* (International Bureau of Weights and Measures) in France changed the way scientists define exact mass of a kilogram and three other units.[272]

All of this means that Tiller reduced the normally very high improbability of exchanging a selected state for another, less improbable one. Via his intention, he created a new world where phenomena, usually inaccessible to our ordinary senses, are so strongly exaggerated that they can be observed as easily as ordinary events in a physics lab. Everything was right for a miracle. All that the system needed was a nudge in a direction by changing probabilities. Anomalous became commonplace. He created more. He *became* more, and becoming means evolving. Science, for Tiller, is a path to self-knowledge. Science and Spirit are a necessary unity.

Any confusion about potentiality and actuality can be eradicated if we admit that our Universe is open to organizing input from elsewhere, including through us. The paradox of nothing causing anything is not a problem with the real world. It is a problem with the assumptions we make when we try to model phenomena.

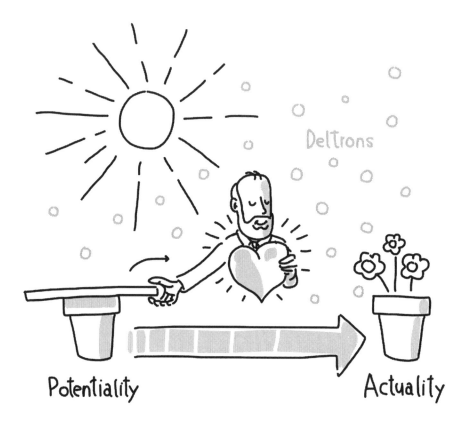

Potentiality

Actuality

[50]
"We can reach for the stars."
The Universe in a Single Atom

Since Paul Dirac first introduced the idea of the physical vacuum, it has remained enigmatic. Science has many questions for this most abundant aspect of our Universe. For one thing, it isn't really "empty." To get an idea of the latent energy density contained in the vacuum, we can take a hydrogen atom. If we blow up the hydrogen atom to the size of a football stadium, at the center of the empty stadium would be the nucleus the size of a marble! The electron would be whizzing way out at the edge of the football stadium. What is between the nucleus and electron? Empty space, the vacuum. Now, technically, there may be some electromagnetic fields, but there is no physical stuff.

John Archibald Wheeler of Princeton University calculated the latent potential energies in the physical vacuum at 10^{94} grams per cubic centimeter of physical space.[273] That is ten with ninety-four zeroes after it, an unimaginably large number. A single hydrogen atom's vacuum space has latent energy that exceeds, by a trillion times, all the energy of matter and "stuff" contained in our cosmos to a radius of fifteen billion light years from Earth! The space of a single hydrogen atom has enough potential energy to sustain the entire Earth and its inhabitants for millennia.

The question is, how do we harness this resource? In his paper "What Are Subtle Energies?" Tiller writes: "We must be able to produce excitations in the vacuum. To perform such a feat, it is necessary to [influence] the Dirac sea such that more constructive interference exists between the wave functions of this virtual level of reality. To date, the one field present in our armory of fields that has been determined to control the phase of the quantum potential is the magnetic vector potential. Since the latent energy potential of one cubic centimeter of vacuum is so huge, it may be not too difficult to 'tilt' the situation a little."[274]

Tiller's physics indicates that we interact with the vacuum all the time to different degrees. By practicing inner quietude and honing focused, powerful intention, we influence the vacuum to a higher level. Tillerian physics is consistent with Spiritual master Vimala Thakar's commentary: "You cannot live without action [intention], even for a minute. You cannot live without the interplay; it is the nature of Life. The [*Bhagavad*] *Gita* says those who offer their actions to the Divine are really sending back the energies to the Cosmos from which they came. They are getting united to the source of Life, the source of all energies. And where is that Divine, that ultimate reality? It is contained in the emptiness of space. In the emptiness of space there are innumerable energies. The energies emanating from you are dedicated to that. They return there."[275]

Mankind's potential for creativity and innovation is inexhaustible. Our species will evolve to greater heights. We have the capacity to reach the stars, and if we have only touched the face of the moon, our intention in this direction are very new.

Similarly, the exploration of inner space, the heart and mind of man, is also only at the barest beginnings.

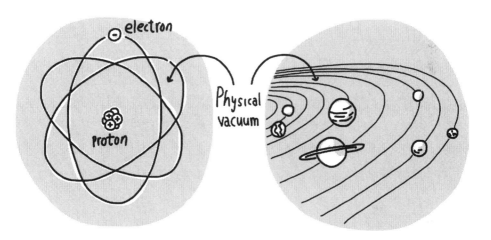

[51]
"Brighten the corner where you are."
You Are the Difference Maker

Tiller says: "We know when a group of humans meditate together, pray together, they create a field—they are raising the symmetry of the space. They are 'pumping' space. When they leave the room, it starts to decay. It is 'metastable.' Then they come back the next day, before it's fully decayed and pump it up a little higher and again, higher still the next day, next week, next month, next year. That's how people have created sacred spaces around the globe. We've all experienced [something special] walking into those spaces."

As we evolve in intention and create our new common ground of experience, sacred spaces assist us on this contemplative and meditative path. Throughout history, mankind has taken pilgrimages to sacred spaces all over Earth. During my research in London, I often spent my lunchtimes in the great space of the Westminster Abbey. I can use my senses to describe Westminster Abbey: the pulpit, stained-glass windows, the fragrance of incense, the high ceilings. But when I close my eyes, the feeling remains. No sight, no sound, no touch. It disappears into me.

A space need not be grand. A physics lab will do, or even deep inside a cave. If you venture to Rishikesh at the foot of the high Himalayas, on the banks of the sacred Ganges river, you find one of the most sacred spaces on Earth. There is no signpost, no writing or announcement. You walk down a short dirt path to the entrance of a cave. It is no ordinary cave. It is the cave of Sage Vashishtha, the teacher of the Hindu God Lord Rama. You enter the semidarkness, which, like a huge magnetic field, pulls you in. The dark, austere cave has no writing, paintings, inscriptions, or symbols, yet it has a field that has endured for more than five thousand years. The interior is exquisite, serene, peaceful beyond all understanding. You feel a sublime "radiation" of the very space, its rocky walls, and its ground. It is metastable, far from equilibrium for centuries! Intention so powerful, we feel the effects today. Can there be a more excellent gift? There is no material stuff, no relics left behind. Here is a different kind of power. Not one of force, but altogether different. Humans have such power. We can grow into such a state.

I am a great believer in the living presence of the past. To arrive here, in Rishikesh, is to enter one of those thrilling places on Earth where the ancient past still exists alongside the modern world. The sublime quality of the Vashishtha cave will likely continue, if history is any guide.

Some of the hugely conditioned exalted spaces I have visited are:
- Tiller laboratories, Payson, Arizona, US (closed at the time of this writing)
- Westminster Abbey, London, UK
- National Shrine of Our Lady of Good Help, New Franken, Wisconsin, US
- St. Joseph's Oratory, Montreal, Canada
- Basilica of Sainte-Anne-de-Beaupré, Quebec City, Canada
- Sanctuary of Saint Pio of Pietrelcina, San Giovanni Rotondo, Italy
- Ashram of the Saint Jalaram Bapa, Virpur, India
- Ashram of Swami Ram Dulare, Madhavpur, India
- Spaces hosting the Buddha's relics tour

- The Gompa (temple) of the Kurukulla Center for Tibetan Buddhist Studies, Boston, Massachusetts, US

So, brighten the corner where you are:
- Pump your intention into your home or office.
- The higher your consciousness, the more concentrated your intention and more powerfully you can condition your space. Consciousness beats lifestyle or any self-improvement tactics.
- To reveal higher levels of consciousness, transcend the lower levels by dropping the barriers to the essence of that which you are, which is Love. This is the essential work to realizing higher consciousness.

Tiller says: "You are being assisted by the great Unseen." His laboratory became a sacred space, for he created an intention statement that invited and called upon God. Tiller created an intimate and extraordinary rapport with God and a mind saturated with God. He knows only faith and possibility and joy without doubt. And he was victorious in building himself, showing that humans can do marvelous deeds, and building the bridge so that his fellow man may cross to the other side.

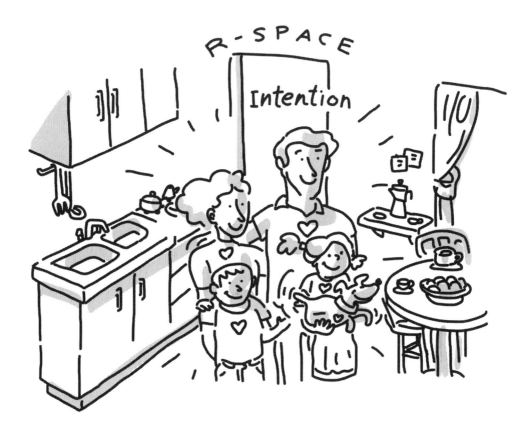

[52]
"Mankind is evolving to adepts, masters, and avatars by the tool of intention."
Become *Homo universalis*

Tiller says: "Generally, what happens if we meditate, we go deep into the silence within, we create new information in ourselves, build it into ourselves; that's called inner-work, and we become more and more coherent. Our real work is to use intention more, create more, and thereby evolve to Adepts, Masters, and Avatars! As you rise in consciousness, your protoplasm is very different. Your body may not decay after death. This has been shown by the incorruptible saints time and time again."

In 2016, I traveled to the sanctuary of the great saint Padre Pio of San Giovanni Rotondo, Italy. It was stunning to behold him, his head cloaked in his monk's habit, the skin and face perfect. As I gazed at his serene face through the glass case, I felt as though Father Pio might wake up any moment and say hello to me. Yet, he had died nearly fifty years prior, on September 23, 1968. His body is incorruptible, meaning, amazingly, that it does not decompose. Millions of people visit his hermitage annually, and thousands of miracles have been attributed to Father Pio.

British economist E. F. Schumacher has written of saints like Father Pio:

> At this supra-human level, [Father Pio] found liberation from constraints that operate at the level of ordinary humanity—limits imposed by space and time, by the needs of the body, and the by the opaqueness

of the computer-like mind. His example illustrates the paradoxical truth that such higher powers cannot be acquired by any kind of conquest conducted by the human personality; only when the striving for "power" has entirely ceased and been replaced by a certain transcendental longing often called the Love of God, may they, or may they not, be "added unto you."[276]

We started our journey across the bridge with Psalm 104:5: "Who laid the foundations of the earth, that it should not be removed forever." Psalm 104:5 is correct, just not in the sense the sixteenth century church had it. Man can be the center of the cosmos, not in an egotistical way, but in the likeness of the Creator. Tiller provides an apropos metaphor:

> "If we look at a light bulb—let's say it's a hundred-watt light bulb—it gives some light, but not a lot of light, and the reason it's not a lot of light is because the photons that come out of the light bulb every second are not in phase with each other and so they interfere. It's called destructive interference. So, there's only a little bit of net light that is given by the hundred-watt light bulb. If you could arrange those photons, the same number coming out per second, if you arrange them to be in phase with each other then, the temperature at the surface of that light bulb with the same number of photons per second coming out would probably be about ten times the surface of our Sun. That is what humans are. Humans are at a place where they're mostly incoherent,

and that's why they have to develop coherence within themselves."[277]

Tiller's metaphor speaks to what many contemporary teachers have made clear of humankind's new promising identity. These messages I bring to you, from the red rocks of Sedona, from the farmlands of the upper Midwest in Wisconsin, and from Shiva's abode in Rajasthan, India, I am thrilled with the consistency, as though I was being provided code words.

> "Humankind evolved from *Homo erectus* to *Homo sapiens* and now is evolving to *Homo spiritus*."
> —David R. Hawkins[278]

> "Man is maturing into *Homo illumine*."
> —Endeavor Academy for *A Course in Miracles*[279]

> "Mankind will evolve to *Homo universalis*. This will happen in your lifetime."
> —Vimala Thakar[280]

Through his target experimental protocol, Tiller has given us the scientific counterpart of a photographic theme that could be called a God's-eye view, like the camera looking straight down from a great height. If the universe is infinite, then even Copernicus would have had to agree that the stage on which you stand is the center of that universe. If the Universe is vastly incomprehensible, then even Descartes would surely have conceded that Tiller's labors were far from superfluous and given his approval of the application of the laws of heat and work that could finally be tested in the laboratory. As we let Tiller's revolutionary results sink in, we're able to see who Tiller is and, better still, who we may become.

This process of becoming is urgent for, around the globe, it seems fear is dividing us by color, creed, sexuality, and more. A bridge provides an apt, hopeful, portending image of human potential, for it joins rather than separates. This bridge expresses the fundamental bonds that exist within and between all human beings. It is functional and symbolic. This bridge will stand the test of time, but we must carry on the work and become builders and engineers in our lives, remembering that *Homo dubitat* and *Homo illumine* are two characters who shape our past and shape us into our future. We have done the work on the bridge's structure: we know why this whole thing works. No matter how the *Homo dubitat* among and within us protests and tinkers, the bridge remains strong. It remains yours and mine. We are creators!

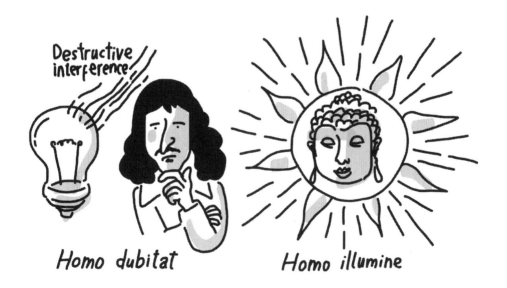

Destructive interference

Homo dubitat   *Homo illumine*

AFTERWORD

Any writer will tell you: You expose yourself through words. To paraphrase Ernest Hemingway, one bleeds at the keyboard. When it came right down to it, I was uneasy about writing this bridge-book because of one simple reason: my lack of formal education in physics. I was terrified of messing things up. Nothing like this book had been done before. After all, I'm not an engineer (not even close). It's hard to drown out these incessant inner noises.

A second reason for my uneasiness was it's not easy to write about the life of Tiller and his contributions to scientific evolution and human thought in the short span of a book like this. In fact, it is not easy to write about any of the luminaries, the giants in science, that I have been writing about. Each one of them has been an extraordinary individual, and the new information each discovered for science and mankind's forward thrust needs deep study and investigation.

Day after day, whether I found myself in Minnesota, California, Arizona, Kenya, or Singapore, between clinics and over lunch hours, I discovered, tossed out, and rejected ideas, only to rediscover them and understand how they helped build my bridge. I endured frozen computers, lost many months of work in a terrifying blinking second due to my ineptness with using writing software programs, dragged around volumes of out-of-print physics books, and spent an inordinate amount of time in libraries.

For my bridge engineering, I had to dive into many concepts, from astronomy to consciousness and the brain, complexities of water (which gave me a new respect for this precious resource), laws of thermodynamics, information and entropy, gauge symmetries and particle physics, the magnetic monopole, and others. What's more, I had to link them in one long structure. In the building phase, I kept the company of savants: the incomparable biologist and thermodynamicist Harold Morowitz, biologist Lyall Watson, medical doctor Lewis Thomas, naturalist Loren Eiseley, and physicist James Trefil. Each inspired me to look at the scientific data before me and reinforced comprehension.

I consider this book as a work in progress, akin to a status report, of where we are in intention research and Information Medicine. Some will complain about my choice for the ideas (the fifty-two "bricks") and how I approached my engineering goals for this book. I make no apology for this. I would say *Bridging Science and Spirit* is a significant and meaningful step. The writing itself was like building a bridge. It was a continual search for the word that would fit in my mind, in the ideas, on the page. As the bridge builder, I erected my structure one brick and pillar at a time until I reached the far end at the opposite bank. If I didn't build it, it wouldn't be there. So I looked at my pile of bricks, of ideas, picked the one that looked like it would fit the best, and put it in.

Tiller discovered in the course of his target experiments the harmful effects of ambient electromagnetic fields (EMF) on biological enzymes and the fruit fly. Although an important topic, it was beyond the scope of this work. I don't have an answer to how to reduce EMF exposure, but I feel a general awareness will go some way toward that goal.

In the new Tiller world, thermodynamics is no longer just an "old" science about heat and work. It is about the deep structure of the concepts contained in thermodynamics; not numbers but processes, transformations, symmetries. This radical view of how humans are connected to universal laws and contribute to the observable phenomena changes the face of consciousness research. Tillerian physics makes it more general and more powerful. Tiller's science helped me as a doctor to understand the importance of "doing all levels" and how spirituality strengthens conventional medicine. These new views were congruent with the way I really wanted to practice medicine. Mark's case report was a revelation to me of the power of Tiller's method. Such a joy crept into me as his suffering lifted.

Tiller's revolutionary science invites us to think about bigger ideas. We have a way to start the second Copernican-scale revolution. We're going to have to figure out how to make Tillerian physics something viable, to make this idea of creating conditioned spaces something we can trust. What else can we do with Tillerian science if it is shown to work consistently? Imagine IHDs for multiple projects in parallel, like lasers sending coherent information for beneficial outcomes. We can start it by creating systems in schools, libraries, nonprofits. It could be a practical proposition. It means people gathering for a common purpose of creating intention information for beneficial uses; it means expert imprinters. It is summoning our individual and collective consciousness. I am reminded of that most marvelous biblical teaching in Matthew 18:20: "Where two or three are gathered together in my name, there am I in the midst of them."

The bridge is constructed, but it isn't completed. If Information Medicine is anything to go by, then I can imagine other industries and endeavors that can be enhanced: thousands of businesses, wellness centers, YWCA, YMCA, and enormous cost savings. It's not too hard to imagine. Jobs of all kinds—and a pumped-up consciousness means a whole new humanity! The feeling of possibility come AI or whatever. All the conditioned spaces and the signs and symbols of a peaceful race, of abundance. We are entering a new phase in history. It's a terrific beginning.

I am still very much a conventional practitioner, doing all the necessary diagnostic analysis and routinely looking to RCTs and evidence-based medicine. However, I seldom use a computer during an interaction, instead preferring the old-fashioned way of a notepad and a pen, sketching medical concepts and reasoning for my patients as they share their information with me and ask questions. Together, we create new information that supports both conventional and complementary and integrative medicine. I routinely "prescribe" energetic therapies like qigong, tai chi, and yoga, and periodically teach guided meditation on a one-on-one basis during an office visit. The Arthritis Foundation® has an excellent tai chi program, among many exercise programs for people with chronic arthritis.[281]

Development of optimal Information Medicine for prevention, personalized care, optimization, and augmentation requires close collaboration between physicists and doctors. Such an interface presents a complex, important, and exciting challenge. Many modern health problems could benefit from Information Medicine: PTSD, neonatal care, cancer wards, and more.

Many readers will wonder about the Buddha's sacred relics. A statue of Maitreya Buddha is being constructed in Kushinagar, India. This statue will house the holy relics to broadcast and radiate unconditional Loving-kindness information of the Buddha Masters throughout the world.[282]

Tiller's wish is "to continue working." Despite being a nonagenarian, he shows no indication of being burned out. He is still imprinting

IHDs, now to reduce crime rates in a major metropolitan US city. If his intention information is anything to go by, it is over 600 on the Hawkins map of consciousness. *Yowza.* It has the juice to make a difference.

Now time to sign off and travel to that sublime space in Rajkot, India, containing the archives of spiritual teacher Vimala Thakar, to kneel at the feet of her legacy, for Vimalaji has proclaimed that we are becoming *Homo universalis.*

ACKNOWLEDGMENTS

Professor William "Bill" and Jean "Jeannie" Tiller for their commitment and dedication to finding the Truth. What mentors! John Gregory "Greg" Fandel and the late Walter Dibble. You have all shown me the power of Love to serve mankind via scientific endeavors. Dr. Tiller, you and Jeannie have truly united the complementary pathways of science (Logos) and spirituality (Mythos). Tillerian physics can quicken mankind's ascent to higher levels of consciousness. I hope my bridge has done a small service to help send your message along.

This book is filled with the power of other people's intentions. Let me tell you about some of them.

My special thanks to Reverend Bill Roberts of the Logos Center, Scottsdale, Arizona. You recognize the power of Tillerian physics operating behind-the-scenes in every prayer and intention. And your sense of humor, well, it cracks me up! You beam deltrons far and wide from the Tiller Institute in Arizona.

To Douglas Matzke, PhD, thanks for demonstrating the power of subtle energy with spoon bending. I am still practicing.

My salutations sent "remotely" to Patricia "Patty" Cyrus, for your remote viewing expertise. Simply incredible.

Michael Kohane, PhD, you did the early "crazy" experimental work to test intention and enzyme function and creating the conditions for happier fruit flies! You reminded me to heed Dr. Tiller's advice to "go to the source" and verify scientific nomenclature. The chapter on zero-point energy is the result of your reminder to stay rigorous to the original meaning of physical definitions. By going back to the source, I could finally release my attachment to the notion that zero-point energy was underpinning consciousness and intention effects. And besides, it's very cold at -273 °C.

Suzy Miller, author of *Awesomism!*, you are awesome indeed. You were the crucial bridge to families of children diagnosed with autism. You could both "hear" what the children asked for and connect with Dr. Tiller. Your and Dr. Tiller's work forever changed my limited perception of children who seemed to have no hope. My profound thank you for opening my eyes.

Dr. Gabriele Hilberg, you've taken on a most-pressing modern problem of loneliness with the rare gift of unconditional lovingness. Need I say more?

Daniel Harner, PhD, and Anthony "Todd" Welch, my buddies on Thursdays. Daniel, your doctoral thesis brought home for me the immensity of what had quietly unfolded in healing autism and loneliness. It has been my honor to be on your team during the preparation of your doctoral thesis. Todd, my friend on the pathway of evolving more in consciousness. Your questions for Dr. Tiller during our Thursday meetings deepened my comprehension.

Special gratitude to Patricia "Pat" Mackay and Charles Begin of Edmonton, Canada, for their untiring information gathering about the change in consciousness of participants during the Information Medicine broadcasts. You both went above and beyond to deliver, and as a result we have a more profound knowledge about the dynamics of the Unseen working with us and through us.

Donese Worden, NMD, and Barry Goldstein, thank you for your passion for Tiller's work. You both "get it."

Professor Fran Grace, PhD, of the University of California, Redlands, in your masterpiece *The Power of Love: A Transformed Heart Changes the World,* you had the heart and courage to bridge science and Spirit.[283] Thank you for your friendship. You "get it."

Professor Hope Umansky, PhD, of the California Institute of Human Science, Encinitas, California, for giving me a chance to share about Tillerian physics to graduate students who want to understand science in the greater context of consciousness. CIHS fulfills the mission of uniting science and Spirit admirably.[284]

Cynthia "Cindy" Reed, RN, PhD, you had the inspiration to recognize the potential in Tillerian physics and conduct the first intention broadcast to alleviate depression and anxiety while at Holos University, Missouri. Boy, Cindy, you've helped open the floodgates and smash the ceiling of conventional medical care! To Steven Lamer, MD, thank you for lifting me by sending your out-of-the-blue text during one of my bleakest and most uncertain moments in my writing attempts to construct the bridge. Your unexpected message means that you and I are entangled in the field of reciprocal space.

Jackie Clowes, MD, PhD, of the Guthrie Clinic, Sayre, Pennsylvania, and Mary Jurisson, MD, of the Mayo Clinic, Rochester, Minnesota, thank you for your marvelous discussions around physics, healing, and subtle energies. Jackie, you are a bridge to this finished work, always encouraging me to: "Keep going. Work hard on your book." Mary, you bring the gift of tai chi by teaching medical doctors and increasing awareness of this important subtle energy therapy for our colleagues.

Master Chunyi Lin of Spring Forest Qigong Healing Center, Minneapolis, Minnesota,[285] your gift of teaching people from around the world about the power of their intention and subtle energies is awesome. I salute you. Professor Yang Yang, PhD, of Taiji Training, who taught Yang style tai chi in Rochester, Minnesota, to newbie practitioners like me.

Steven Tonsager, LAc, and Ardith, in your clinic, you create the conditions for healing on all levels.[286] Accessing new information from higher domains of R-space field benefits your clients' healing; it also speeds along medicine in the near future toward informational healing.

James "Jim" Seidl, JD, for being an active supporter of the unfolding adventure of Tillerian physics. Your faith and trust in Dr. Tiller and me mean so much. Thank you always.

Deanna Won, Colonel, USAF (Ret), and Patricia "Trish" Lynch, you both have remarkable personal stories of physical healing when modern medicine gave up all hope. You are thermodynamic pumper-uppers! Trish, may your new book, *Letters to God: Transforming Crisis into Consciousness,* help everyone use their gifts of intention and evolve faster even in the face of chronic illness.[287]

Deepest thanks to my teammate and medical assistant extraordinaire Barbara King, for holding down the fort at the clinic. My patients who show me the power of intention and the power of the human spirit in the face of chronic illness, thank you.

George Munoz, MD, founder of the OASIS Arthritis and Osteoporosis Clinic, Miami, Florida, and Jose Pando, MD, of the Delaware Arthritis Center—thank you both for being pioneers in complementary and integrative medicine for rheumatology, for recognizing the physical body's energetic and informational systems, and for continually checking in via D-space emails and phone calls to see if "Nisha is OK." I am happy that we are entangled via the R-space information superhighways.

My gratitude to Professor Randy Horwitz, MD, PhD, of the University of Arizona, Tucson, who loved the story of Information Medicine when we presented together at the international American College of Rheumatology scientific meetings.

Professor Kathi Kemper, MD, MPH, of Ohio State University's Department of Pediatrics, Executive Director, Center for Integrative Health and Wellness, and author of *Authentic Healing: A Practical Guide for Caregivers,* you are an amazing role model for me, combining the best of traditional medicine with your loving intention in using therapeutic touch to heal children under your care. Your insatiable curiosity about Tillerian physics, I hope, will be answered or rewarded. Thanks also to Robert Sheeler, MD, of the Next Level Clinic, Scottsdale, and John Kolstoe, MD, rheumatologist in the Sanford Health system, Northern Minnesota, who bring the integrative principle of "doing all levels" to their daily work at the bedside.

My deepest Love and appreciation to Venerable Kyabje Lama Zopa Rinpoche for illuminating the world by way of the Maitreya Project's Buddha's sacred relic tour. By doing so, you helped create the conditions to quicken mankind's evolution to *Homo illumine.* I dedicate this work to Rinpoche's long life for the benefit of all sentient beings. May wisdom and Loving-kindness spread throughout the world. Venerable Roger Sumden, Paula Chichester, Victoria Coleman (née Ewart), Dana Lissy, Dekyi Lee Oldershaw, Gandhi Megena, Andrea Bridger, Cristian Cowan, Amanda Karg, Amanda Russell, and all of the Maitreya Buddha relic tour. Thank you to my dear friends Nancy and Thupten Dadak of Minneapolis. You know why. Special "Tashi Delek" to The Gyuto Wheel of Dharma Monastery, Minneapolis, Minnesota.

Joseph Gallenberger, PhD, of the Monroe Institute, in your book *Inner Vegas Adventure* you show psychoenergetic science at work at the craps table![288] Most of all, Dr. Joe you kept me grounded in the power of my heart and helped me to experience love's mysterious ways even in a casino in Las Vegas. Love knows no bounds, nor does it judge. Our intentions matter. You and Elena help people to experience their inner power in such a tangible way.

Thanks to the marvelous Sivananda Ashram, Nassau, Bahamas, for inviting the Tiller Institute to share Tillerian science for the benefit of all seekers. I feel fortunate and grateful to be included in the Ashram's special family.

Dr. Todd Hoover ("Vidyacharya") and Lisa Hoover ("Acharya Ma Punyashila") of Life Mission, Mebane, North Carolina, I will never forget the love with which you both taught me about Vedic life and resurrecting the teachings of Mahadeva, Lord Shiva Lakulish. Lord Lakulish reminds us that our ultimate reality is beyond space and time. Jai Bhagwan! Shreyas Karia of Vimal Prakashan Trust, Rajkot, India, for making available the archived teachings of Shree Vimala Thakar. Vimalaji ascended to Avatar and by magnificent approach to living fearlessly, she showed us the ideals of *Homo universalis.*

To my fellow authors, Susan Flint and Raj Rajkumar, of South India, who beat me to publishing their first book, *Artificial Intelligence: The Final Dominion.*[289] To psychoenergetic superstars Stanislav and Helen O'Jack, for conducting early research into subtle energy instrument sensitization. To personal development consultant Anya Sophia Mann for making available to me archived Tiller interviews from her radio show "Quantum Alchemy."

Marci Reiss, licensed clinical social worker, founder & president, Inflammatory Bowel Disease (IBD) Support Foundation, AGA Academy of Educators Los Angeles, California, for your zeal for rigorous conventional science combined with spirituality. Michael Billauer, DC, of the Los Angeles Wellness Institute, and Edward Wagner, DC, of Wagner Holistic Center in Pacific Palisades, California, I always remember your mantra of "get fixed." Becky Carrol, PhD, for your joyous spirit and asking to be shown the main bridge points to understand Dr. Tiller. Becky, I hope this book helps you!

Raj and Jay Manek. Neal Mody. Arjun Paurana. Professor Prem Saint, PhD. My friend Lynne Boisineau. Thank you, all.

In illustrating *Bridging Science and Spirit,* Dario Paniagua of Lecco, Italy, said to me: "I want to help you with your book." A shot of deltrons for transforming my basic sketches into designs that brought me joy. *Grazie mille.*

Scottsdale Mustang Public Library, Yorba Linda Public Library, and the central library system of the National University of Singapore.

Tori and the team at Eye Comb Editors, for your editorial expertise. Your editing made me dig deeper. The rambling bridge became tighter, the foundations sturdier, thanks to you all.

BONUS SECTION

The Tiller Intention Academy
Creating Your Intention

1) Meditate.
2) Determine what your intention is.
3) Gather all details related to your intention.
4) Write down your intention.
   Remember, you're creating new information.
5) Make the intention informed and succinct.
6) Revise freely and often until you feel peaceful.
   If using an IHD, include location of your imprinted device and location of the recipient.
7) Visualize your intention with God as your partner.
8) Ask to be shown the Truth.
9) Repeat for life.
10) Become *Homo Spiritus*

The Tiller Intention Academy
Imprinting Your Intention

1) Choose a quiet place and time.
2) Meditate and connect together through the heart using your own words/methods.
3) Call on your chosen helper/deity and connect with them.
4) Feel the emotion - Remember that intention comes from your emotion domain. Pump joyful emotion into your space.
5) Read the intention aloud.
6) Take the intention inside and visualize the outcome.
7) Be completely present and open to the process.
8) Visualize the intention being imprinted into the device.
9) When you feel the process is complete say, "Thy will be done."
10) Let go completely (of the intention).
11) Check with helper/deity for confirmation.
12) Seal and protect your IHD using your own words.
   You may wrap the IHD in aluminum foil for further protection.

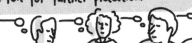

APPENDIX 1
Patricia Cyrus's remote viewing sketch

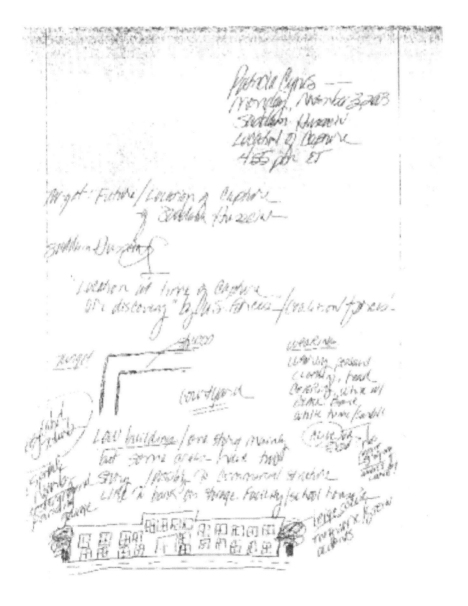

APPENDIX 2

In muscle testing, a two-person team can test "information" to determine whether a statement has the integrity of truth; that is, whether it is correct (yes, or muscle is strong) or incorrect (not yes, or muscle is weak). The "information" is in the form of a declarative statement, and while one team member holds the statement in mind, the other's muscle—commonly the deltoid muscle of the upper arm, is tested for strength. The "information" may be delivered verbally or nonverbally by the tester who holds the statement in mind while pressing down on the testing partner's outstretched arm. If the "information" is not true, then the deltoid muscle becomes weak instantaneously. "Information" that is in harmony allows the person's deltoid to remain strong. An individual can also test the level of truth by testing muscle strength of his or her thumb and opposing index finger, in the "O" ring configuration while holding the information in mind.

APPENDIX 3

Dr. William A. Tiller's Intention Statement for Self-Compassion Information Medicine Broadcast:

(Note: This broadcast to increase self-compassion measures (calibrates) at a consciousness level of 545 out of 1,000 on the Hawkins Map of Consciousness, on which 200 is neutral and 600 is enlightenment).

- The purpose of this intention is to strengthen with a compassionate heart our experience of a shared humanity.

- While recognizing the uniqueness of each human being, we deeply acknowledge our common bond.

- All human beings are indivisible and interdependent parts of the Eternal Being and therefore ARE the infinite perfection of all creation.

- By shifting from identification with our limited form to knowing ourselves as Eternal Being, we dissolve our ego-centric feelings of unworthiness, isolation, and being separate.

- It is safe to allow the LOVE of ALL THAT IS to fully express itself in all aspects of your conscious and unconscious existence. You may now allow any and all thought patterns, grievances, and wounds, which are obscuring the experience of Universal Love, to gently fall away.

- Knowing ourselves as ALL THAT IS spontaneously gives rise to kindness, compassion, and acceptance for both self and others.

GLOSSARY

A

absolute zero: A temperature of -273 °C; the coldest temperature theoretically possible to attain.

adaequatio: Term used by British economist E. F. Schumacher to represent the qualifications of a scientist as well as tools that are adequate and up to the task of scientific inquiry.

Ankylosing spondylitis: An uncommon inflammatory arthritis affecting the spine, joint tissues, and tendons.

asymptotically: Coming into consideration as a variable approaches a limit, usually infinity.

B

Bénard convection: A type of natural convection whereby air temperature oscillations in a room are caused by a density inversion in the air: warm air at the floor and cooler air at the ceiling. In a gravity field, the buoyancy and upwelling of less-dense air from the heated bottom layer spontaneously organizes into a regular pattern of convection cells.

Bit: The objective measurement of the amount of information contained in a message and consists of 0's and 1's from the binary number system. The binary code assigns a pattern of binary digits, known as bits, to each character in a message thereby compressing it and sending it with perfect accuracy.

Boltzmann's constant (k): 1.38×10^{-23} joules/Kelvin.

C

Cartesian: Pertaining to the philosophy of René Descartes.

conjugate: as noun: a mathematical value or entity having a reciprocal relation with another; as adjective: to couple, connect, or relate.

cogito: Consciousness. Latin word meaning "I think."

D

D-space: (Direct-space): Tiller's term for spacetime.

deltrons: To solve the dilemma of a massive particle traveling slower than the velocity of light interacting with a wave component traveling faster than the velocity of speed of light, Tiller postulates the existence of a moiety from the domain of emotion, which he calls the "deltron." Deltrons link the D-space (which is subluminal, slower than the speed of light) and R-space (superluminal, faster than the speed of light) dimensions.

dissipative: Throwing off of heat (as waste) to the surroundings by a system.

differential equations: Results of these equations give functions at each point on a curve. The Schrodinger equation is an example of a second-order differential equation. The solution at each point on a wave gives the probability of the particle at that position.

dowsing: A type of divination usually employed to locate ground water, buried metals, oil reserves, and many other objects without the use of scientific apparatus.

E

electromagnetic wave: Transmits energy through electric and magnetic fields. The carrier particle is photons. Electromagnetism has a spectrum of wavelengths: radio, infrared, visible colors, X-rays, etc.

electron volt (eV): By definition, it is the amount of energy required to move an electron across a potential difference of one volt.

energy: Quantity that dictates potential of change by being exchanged. The accepted definition is "power to do work." It isn't energy per se, but the *flow* of energy through a system that does work.

entanglement: Connectivity between parts of a system separated in physical distance.

entropy: It is a quantity that measures the disorder of a system and can be applied to any situation in which there are multiple possibilities. Entropy is also a lack of information about a system in question.

equilibrium: Implies a state of balance. In an equilibrium state, there are no unbalanced potentials (or driving forces) within the system. In thermodynamics, a system is said to be in equilibrium where there is no change in macroscopic property and the system never changes to any other state spontaneously.

Evidence-Based Medicine (EBM): Data from clinical trials used as evidence to inform doctors' decisions.

F

field: Magnetic, electric, gravity—a means of transmitting a force at a distance. Force and field are related. All fundamental particles have associated fields. Particles act as carriers.

Fourier transform: Mathematical operation which converts an equation with the variations in distance and/or time into one with the variations in spatial or temporal frequency.

G

gauge theory: Relates to the effects of symmetry transformations on physics equations, which can be local or global and are important to the success of mathematics in physics. Maxwell's electromagnetic field theory has gauge symmetry. In general, gauge theories were constructed to relate the properties of the four known fundamental forces of nature (gravity, electromagnetism, the strong nuclear force, and the weak nuclear force) to the various symmetries of nature.

Gedankenexperiment: A thought experiment made famous by Albert Einstein.

geocentric theory: Theory that the Sun revolves around the Earth. This was premise of the astronomy of Claudius Ptolemy and was accepted by the Catholic Church in the sixteenth century.

Gibbs free energy: Dictates what spontaneous processes occur in nature, releasing energy that can be harnessed for performing work. In thermodynamics, one of the most important quantities is the Gibbs free energy per unit volume, denoted G, of a material. It varies in magnitude with pressure, temperature, and chemical concentration as its main intensive variables. Secondary variables are electric, magnetic, and gravitational fields. Tiller physics expands contributions to G from information and reduced entropy of the physical vacuum.

Granny effect: Connectivity between parts of a system separated in distance and time. Effects are due to subtle energy magnetic wave information entanglement effects.

H

hypothesis: Theory that can be experimentally tested.

heliocentric theory: Theory that Earth revolves around the Sun, put forward by Nicolaus Copernicus in 1543.

Higgs boson: Particle named after Scottish physicist Peter Higgs. Gives particles their mass by transfer of bosons and interaction with the Higgs field.

Higgs field: Carried by the Higgs boson; subatomic fundamental particles such as quarks and leptons are heavier because they are slowed while traversing the Higgs field. As an analogy, imagine dropping a bead into a glass of water versus an empty glass filled with air. It will take longer for the bead to drop to the bottom as it traverses through water than air. It is as if the bead has more mass in water and gravity takes longer to pull it through the "field" of liquid. The bead will be slowed even more if dropped into a glass of molasses. The Higgs field slows down other particles, effectively giving them a mass.

Homo dubitat ((man/being who doubts)): New information (term) created by the author based on her practiced use of skepticism in scientific endeavors, in accord with a principle of Cartesian logic and investigation.

Homo piger (lazy man/being): New information (term) created by the author to denote traits of the modern sedentary and lazy man.

Homo illumine (self-illumined man/being): Term for future man who is self-illumined.

Homo sapiens (wise man/being): The human with a frontal brain.

Homo spiritus (spiritual man/being): Term used by Dr. David Hawkins, MD, PhD, to denote modern man's evolution to the spiritual man.

Homo universalis (universal man/being): Term used by spiritual teacher Shree Vimalaji Thakar to denote future brotherhood and union of mankind.

I

ion: An atom or molecule with a net electric charge due to the loss or addition of an electron.

information: Fundamental concept that can be given an objective meaning and which has the basic unit of *bit,* a digit whose value is either zero or one. In this book, information of any type is an aspect of thermodynamic free energy and free energy drives all processes in nature.

intention: In this book, intention represents action of consciousness and self-directed mind.

intention host device (IHD): A plastic "black box" with a circuit which has been programmed by humans from a deep meditative state with one specific subtle energy information. It serves as a repository of this information. The specific intention is created to change a particular material property in a given direction and to a given degree.

imprinting: A process whereby humans from a deep meditative state intentionally create a subtle energy field of information that is stored in an object that then serves as a metastable (active) repository of specific information.

K

kinesiology: Muscle testing that accesses the meridian system. It is similar to dowsing phenomena and requires a human.

L

Louie de Broglie: Founder of quantum mechanics and who, at the 1927 Solvay conference, was one of the first to postulate particle-wave duality.

logarithm function: Mathematical technique for simplifying long multiplications. It tells us how to multiply numbers by adding related numbers instead. For example, 1,000 has the exponent notation 103, and the log of the number is 3. The number 100 has the exponent notation 10^2, and the log of the number is 2. The number 0.01 has notation 10^{-2} and log number -2. Similarly, 0.001 has the exponent notation 10^{-3}, and the log number is -3.

light, speed of: *Exactly* 299,792,458 meters per second (186,000 miles per second). The speed of light in a vacuum, commonly denoted *c*, is a universal physical constant.

M

magnetoelectrochemical potential: Expansion of the electrochemical potential by the addition of a magnetic energy term, ΔG^*_{H+}, involving the product of a magnetic charge and a magnetic potential.

Maxwell's equations: A set of four differential equations derived by Scottish physicist James Clerk Maxwell that elegantly and concisely describe classical electromagnetism.

Maitreya Buddha: Name derived from the Sanskrit *maitri,* which means "universal love," who will be the fifth and next Buddha to appear in the world during this "fortunate aeon of one thousand Buddhas."

metastable: System that is excited above ground state.

mirror principle: Mathematical relationship of an inversion (not reflection) mirror kind between substances in D-space and their conjugate quality in R-space.

N

negentropy: Characterized by a reduction in entropy (and corresponding increase in order).

nonequilibrium thermodynamics: System that is not at ground state.

P

phase: The relative shift in wavelength between the peaks of two waves.

phenomenal consciousness: To do with feelings like joy, happiness, sadness, etc.

physical vacuum: The state in which all fields have their lowest possible energy.

psychoenergetic: Encompasses parapsychology and spirituality-related phenomena. Examples include psychokinetics and remote viewing.

Q

qigong: Meditative movement practice related to tai chi.

quantum mechanics: The laws of the sub-atomic world, many of which are counterintuitive but follow mathematical rules.

R

randomized controlled trial (RCT): The gold standard method in medical research to test the effectiveness of a medicine against a dummy (inert) compound in people randomly assigned to either group.

relics: Remains of highly conscious and evolved humans, known as *ringsels* in Tibetan Buddhist traditions, left in the Masters' cremated ashes. Masters' personal effects and clothing may also be considered relics. In the author's experience, relics behave like "imprinted devices" that hold the essence of an enlightened Master, such as unconditional Love. The Loving essence is a form of higher order subtle energy. Christian saints also have relics, whether body relics or possessions.

remote viewing: A mental ability that allows a human to access detailed information concerning a target that is inaccessible to normal senses due to separation in distance or time.

R-space: (Reciprocal space): Reciprocal subspace to spacetime. In R-space, thermodynamic and Maxwell's equations apply to a higher SU(2) gauge state where both electric charges (currents) and magnetic monopoles coexist. In Tillerian physics model, this R-space can be tuned to be responsive to specific intention for a material property change.

S

scalar: A quantity or phenomenon that exhibits magnitude only, with no specific direction, is a scalar. Temperature, for example, is specified by one number and does not depend on direction from a point. This is in contrast to a vector, which has both magnitude and direction.

space conditioning: Enlarged beyond adjustment of usual outer thermodynamic variables of space such as temperature, pressure, chemical concentration and so forth to include inner variables like electromagnetic gauge symmetry state, specific intention, and magnetoelectric contributions. Space conditioning has higher free thermodynamic free energy.

spacetime: Geometric space combined with time in one function in relativity.

steady-state system: An unchanging condition, system, or physical process that remains the same after transformation or change. When you have a chemical mix that has certain properties and the mix retains those properties even after you add a change agent, this is an example of a steady state.

subtle energy: Energies and forces separate from the four fundamental forces (electromagnetism, strong and weak nuclear forces, and gravity). The meridian and chakra systems are subtle energies. In the author's experience, subtle energies can be felt and directed in the body at will through practices such as tai chi, qigong, and Feldenkrais.

subluminal: Slower than the speed of light.

superluminal: Faster than the speed of light.

symmetry: an operation that can be performed on a system that leaves the system invariant.

T

tai chi: Far Eastern wellness and mind–body technique based on ancient martial arts traditions. There are five major lineages, and thousands of forms stem from the basic five.

thermodynamic free energy: This is a quantity (per unit volume or per mole) that defines potential for doing work (if harnessed). This quantity includes both energy and entropy contributions and their dependence on the thermodynamic intensive variables of temperature, pressure, concentration of chemical species, plus electric, magnetic, gravitational fields, etc.

U

unimprinted electronic device (UED): A plastic box with a simple circuit that serves as a control in the Tiller target experiments.

V

vector: A vector has properties of direction and magnitude. Electric fields, magnetic fields, and the gravitational field have vector qualities and require three numbers at a point for complete specification: one is the vector magnitude while the other two are directions from that point relative to some frame of reference. Thus, the vector magnitude at a point varies with direction around that point.

W

wave-particle duality: Behavior, particularly of light, that is sometimes wavelike and at other times like a particle.

Z

zero-point energy (ZPE): Defined as the energies associated with all modes of motion of physical atoms at the temperature of absolute zero (0 K or -273 °C). This includes the electromagnetic light (photon) spectrum in equilibrium with these changing modes.

zero-point field (ZPF): Since electromagnetic energy is proportional to the square of the electromagnetic field, the zero-point field is proportional to the square root of the zero-point energy.

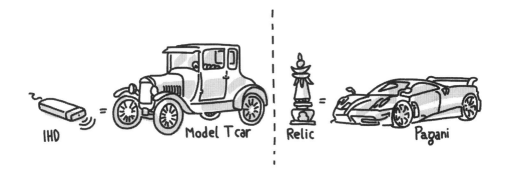

NOTES

Preface

1 William A. Tiller, *Psychoenergetic Science: A Second Copernican-Scale Revolution* (Walnut Creek, CA: Pavior, 2007).

Introduction

2 W. A. Tiller and W. E. Dibble, "Expanding Thermodynamic Perspective for Materials in SU (2) Electromagnetic (EM) Gauge Symmetry State Space: Part 1, Duplex Space Model with Applications to Homeopathy," *Materials Research Innovations* 11, no. 4 (2007): 163–68.

3 David J. Chalmers, "Facing Up to the Problem of Consciousness." *Journal of Consciousness Studies* 2, no. 3 (1995): 200–219.

BRIDGE PILLAR 1: Of Truth and Revolutions: Mankind Is Set Spinning and The Birth of The Miraculous Science

4 Erica Wagner, *Chief Engineer: Washington Roebling, the Man Who Built the Brooklyn Bridge* (New York: Bloomsbury, 2017), Foreword, Kindle edition.

5 Jack Repcheck, *Copernicus' Secret: How the Scientific Revolution Began* (New York: Simon & Schuster, 2007), Epigraph, Kindle edition.

(1) "Copernicus set off a revolution in science."

6 Lewis Thomas, *The Medusa and the Snail: More Notes of a Biology Watcher* (New York: Penguin, 1995), Book Section: A Trip Abroad, Kindle edition.

7 Tiller, *Psychoenergetic Science.*

8 Owen Gingerich, *God's Universe* (Cambridge, MA: Belknap, 2006).

9 Owen Gingerich, *God's Planet* (Cambridge, MA: Harvard University Press, 2014), Chapter 1: Was Copernicus Right? Kindle edition.

10 Gingerich, *God's Planet,* Chapter 1.

11 Gingerich, *God's Planet,* Chapter 1.

12 Dava Sobel, *A More Perfect Heaven: How Copernicus Revolutionized the Cosmos* (London: Bloomsbury, 2012), Chapter 2, Kindle edition.

13 Gingerich, *God's Planet,* Chapter 1.

14 Khan Academy, "Nicolaus Copernicus: A Sun-Centered View of the Universe," *How Did Our View of the Universe Change?* khanacademy.org, accessed March 11, 2019, https://www.khanacademy.org/partner-content/big-history-project/big-bang/how-did-big-bang-change/a/nicolaus-copernicus-bh.

15 Gingerich, *God's Planet,* Chapter 1; Dava Sobel, A More Perfect Heaven, Prelude, Kindle edition.

16 Gingerich, *God's Planet,* Chapter 1.

17 Lisa Rosenbaum, "Resisting the Suppression of Science," *New England Journal of Medicine* 376, no. 17 (2017): 1607–9.

(2) "Descartes's legacy continues to live in modern science."

18 Jacques Maritain, *The Dream of Descartes,* trans. M. L. C. Andison (London: Editions Poetry London, 1946).

19 Genevieve Rodis-Lewis, *Descartes: His Life and Thought* (Ithaca, NY: Cornell University Press, 1999), 17.

20 René *Descartes, Discourse on the Method of Rightly Conducting*

One's Reason and of Seeking Truth in the Sciences (Hamburg, Germany: Tredition Classics, 2011), Book Section: Part I, Kindle edition.

21 Descartes, *Discourse on the Method,* book section: Part VI, Kindle edition.

22 "René Descartes," *Stanford Encyclopedia of Philosophy,* published December 3, 2009, revised January 16, 2014, accessed March 12, 2019, https://plato.stanford.edu/entries/descartes/.

23 Descartes, Dis*course on the Method,* Book Section: Part IV, Kindle edition.

24 Russell Shorto, *Descartes' Bones: A Skeletal History of the Conflict Between Faith and Reason* (New York: Doubleday, 2008), Chapter 1, Kindle edition.

25 Stephen Gaukroger, *Descartes: An Intellectual Biography* (Oxford: Clarendon, 2003).

(3) "Medicine is stuck in chemistry."

26 Shorto, *Descartes' Bones,* Chapter 1, Kindle edition.

27 René Descartes, *Delphi Collected Works of René Descartes* (Delphi Series Seven Book 25, Delphi Classics), book section: Rules for the Direction of the Mind, Rule II, Kindle edition.

28 Descartes, *Discourse on the Method,* Book Section: Part VI, Kindle edition.

29 N. S. Downing et al., "Postmarket Safety Events among Novel Therapeutics Approved by the US Food and Drug Administration Between 2001 and 2010," *Journal of the American Medical Association* 317, no. 18 (2017): 1854–63.

30 James Le Fanu, *The Rise & Fall of Modern Medicine* (London:

Abacus Software, 2014).

31 "What Is a Genome?" Human Genome Project, National Institutes of Health, accessed 19 May 2019, https://www.genome.gov/human-genome-project/Completion-FAQ.

32 "Genetic Similarities of Mice and Men," Genetics 1010, 23andMeBlog, April 20, 2012, accessed January 15, 2019, https://blog.23andme.com/23andme-and-you/genetics-101/genetic-similarities-of-mice-and-men/.

33 Lewis Thomas, *The Medusa and the Snail,* Book Section: The Health Care System, Kindle edition.

34 James Le Fanu, *Too Many Pills: How Too Much Medicine Is Endangering Our Health and What We Can Do About It (*New York: Little, Brown, 2018); The British Museum, "Cradle to Grave," accessed May 1, 2019, http://www.cradletograve.org/.

35 Descartes, *Delphi Collected Works of René Descartes,* Book Section: Rules for the Direction of the Mind, Rule VIII, Kindle edition.

36 Kathi J. Kemper, *Authentic Healing: A Practical Guide for Caregivers* (Minneapolis, MN: Two Harbors Press, 2016); James L. Oschman, *Energy Medicine in Therapeutics and Human Performance* (Edinburgh: Butterworth-Heinemann, 2003); Chunyi Lin and Gary Rebstock, *Born a Healer* (Eden Prairie, MN: Spring Forest, 2003).

37 C. P. West, L. N. Dyrbye, and T. D. Shanafelt, "Physician Burnout: Contributors, Consequences and Solutions," *Journal of Internal Medicine* 283, no. 6 (2018): 516–29.

38 C. Center et al., "Confronting Depression and Suicide in Physicians: A Consensus Statement," *Journal of the*

American Medical Association 289, no. 23 (2003): 3161–66.

39 Astro Teller, *Astro Teller Captain Moonshots,* in *The Tim Ferriss Show.* 2018, Tim Ferriss San Francisco, accessed January 15, 2019, https://www.youtube.com/watch?v=-gJAwCtqaWg.

40 Thomas, *The Medusa and the Snail,* Book Section: Medical Lessons from History, Kindle edition.

41 Barry Marshall, "Helicobacter pylori–A Nobel Pursuit?" *Canadian Journal of Gastroenterology* 22, no. 11 (2008): 895–96.

42 Thomas, *The Medusa and the Snail,* Book Section: Medical Lessons from History, Kindle edition.

(4) "Humans are not just chemistry. They are a mix of energy, information, and spirit."

43 T. C. Clarke, L. I. Black, B. J. Stussman, P. M. Barnes, and R. L. Nahin, "Trends in the Use of Complementary Health Approaches Among Adults: United States, 2002–2012," *National Health Statistics Reports,* no. 79 (2015): 1–16.

44 S. H. Saydah and M. S. Eberhardt, "Use of Complementary and Alternative Medicine among Adults with Chronic Diseases: United States 2002," *Journal of Alternative and Complementary Medicine* 12, no. 8 (2006): 805–812.

45 N. J. Manek et al., "What Rheumatologists in the United States Think of Complementary and Alternative Medicine: Results of a National Survey," *BMC Complementary and Alternative Medicine* 10 (2010): 5.

46 "High Impact Journals: Superfund Research Program," National Institute of Environmental Health Sciences website, accessed January 24, 2019, https://tools.niehs.nih.gov/srp/publications/highimpactjournals.cfm.

47 C. Wang et al., "A Randomized Trial of Tai Chi for Fibromyalgia," *New England Journal of Medicine* 363, no. 8 (2010): 743–54.

48 N. J. Manek and Chunyi Lin, "Qigong," in *Textbook of Complementary and Alternative Medicine,* 2nd edn., ed. Chun-Su Yuan, Eric J. Bieber, and Brent Bauer (Boca Raton, FL: Informa, 2006), 199–210.

49 Erminia Guarneri and Rauni Prittinen King, "Challenges and Opportunities Faced by Biofield Practitioners in Global Health and Medicine: A White Paper," *Global Advances in Health and Medicine* 4, supplement (2015): 89–96.

50 Leon M. Lederman and Christopher T. Hill, *Symmetry and the Beautiful Universe* (Amherst, NY: Prometheus, 2014), Chapter 4: Symmetry, Space, and Time, Kindle edition.

51 Tiller and Dibble, "Expanding Thermodynamic: Part 1," 163–68.

(5) "Subtle energies are not one of the traditional forces in science."

52 William A. Tiller, "A Gas Discharge Device for Investigating Focused Human Attention," *Journal of Scientific Exploration* 4, no. 2 (1990): 255–71.

53 "Townsend Discharge," accessed May 5, 2019, Wikipedia, https://wikivisually.com/wiki/Townsend_discharge.

54 William A. Tiller, "What Are Subtle Energies?" *Journal of Scientific Exploration* 7, no. 3 (1993): 293–304.

55 Jorge Cham and Daniel Whiteson, *We Have No Idea: A Guide to the Unknown Universe* (New York: Penguin, 2017), Chapter 2: What Is Dark Matter? Kindle edition.

56 Cham and Whiteson, *We Have No Idea,* Chapter 2, Kindle edition.

57 Cham and Whiteson, *We Have No Idea,* Chapter 2, Kindle

edition.

58 John Taylor, *Superminds: An Investigation into the Paranormal* (London: Picador, 1976).

59 "John G. Taylor," *Wikipeida,* accessed April 23, 2019, https://en.wikipedia.org/wiki/John_G._Taylor.

(6) "Psychoenergetic science points the way to new possibilities for man."

60 Paul Arthur Schilpp et al., *The Library of Living Philosophers,* ed. P. A. Schilpp *[With autobiographical essays, bibliographies and portraits.]* (Evanston, IL: Northwestern University, 1939), 683.

61 Robert G. Jahn and Brenda J. Dunne, *Margins of Reality: The Role of Consciousness in the Physical World* (Princeton, NJ: ICRL Press, 2009), Kindle edition.

62 Russel Targ and Harold E. Puthoff, *Mind-Reach: Scientists Look at Psychic Abilities* (Charlottsville, VA: Hampton Roads, 2005), Preface to 2004 edition, Kindle edition.

63 Central Intelligence Agency, *DOD Psychoenergetics Program,* DoD (2016), accessed March 15, 2019, https://www.cia.gov/library/readingroom/document/cia=rdp96-00789r002100230001-3.

64 Stephan A. Schwartz, "Finding Saddam Hussein: A Study in Applied Remote Viewing," *EdgeScience,* 2018. https://www.scientificexploration.org/edgescience.

65 Patricia Cyrus (remote viewer) in discussion with the author via email, March 25, 2019.

66 D. E. Graff and Patricia Cyrus, *Perceiving the Future News: Evidence for Retrocausation,* American Institute of Physics (AIP Conference Proceedings, 2017).

67 Lyn Buchanan, *The Seventh Sense: The Secrets of Remote Viewing as Told by a "Psychic Spy" for the U.S. Military* (New York: Paraview Pocket, 2003), Chapter 7, Kindle edition.

68 Paramhansa Yogananda, *Autobiography of a Yogi* (Self-Realization Fellowship, 2017), Chapter 22, Kindle edition.

(7) "The electromagnetic world is complete with the discovery of the Higgs boson."

69 "Lord Shiva Statue Unveiled," CERN bulletin, issue 27/2004 (Meyrin, Switzerland: CERN, 2004), accessed January 30, 2019, https://cds.cern.ch/record/745737/?ln=en.

70 "The Large Hadron Collider," CERN website, accessed January 3, 2019, https://home.cern/science/accelerators/large-hadron-collider.

71 Cham and Whiteson, *We Have No Idea,* Chapter 1, Kindle edition.

72 "Shivanandalahari," by Adishankara Bhagavatpada – English Translation, accessed May 21, 2019, https://shaivam.org/scripture/English-Translation/1433/shivanandalahari-by-adishankara-bhagavatpada-english-translation. The Shivananda Lahari is a devotional hymn composed by Adi Shankaracharya, the eighth-century Advaita philosopher, in praise of Shiva. It literally means Wave of Auspicious Bliss.

BRIDGE PILLAR 2: Mind beyond Brain and Levels of Being

73 Judith Dupre, *Bridges: A History of the World's Most Spectacular Spans* (New York: Running Press, 2017), London Bridge, Kindle edition.

74 Itzhak Bentov, *Stalking the Wild Pendulum: On the Mechanics of*

Consciousness (Rochester, VT: Destiny Books, 1988), Preface, Kindle edition.

(8) "Consciousness is not localized in your brain."

75 "The BRAIN Initiative," National Institutes of Health, accessed March 15, 2019, https://www.braininitiative.nih.gov/.

76 "The NIH Blueprint for Neuroscience Research," National Institutes for Health, accessed March 15, 2019, https://neuroscienceblueprint.nih.gov/.

77 A. W. Yeung, T. K. Goto, and W. K. Leung, "The Changing Landscape of Neuroscience Research, 2006-2015: A Bibliometric Study," *Frontiers in Neuroscience* 11 (2017): 120.

78 Alan Jasanoff, *The Biological Mind: How Brain, Body, and Environment Collaborate to Make Us Who We Are* (New York: Basic Books, 2018), Chapter 4, Kindle edition.

79 Chalmers, "Facing up to the Problem of Consciousness," 200–219.

80 Lyall Watson, *Gifts of Unknown Things: A True Story of Nature, Healing, and Initiation from Indonesia's "Dancing Island"* (Rochester, VT: Destiny Books, 1991), 216.

81 Stuart Hameroff and Roger Penrose, "Consciousness in the Universe: A Review of the 'Orch OR' Theory," *Physics of Life Reviews* 11, no. 1 (2014): 39–78.

82 Emeran Mayer, *The Mind-Gut Connection: How the Hidden Conversation within Our Bodies Impacts Our Mood, Our Choices, and Our Overall Health* (New York: Harper Wave, 2018), Chapter 2: How the Mind Communicates with the Gut, Kindle edition.

83 Eben Alexander, *Into the Afterlife: A Neurosurgeon's Near-*

Death Experience and Spiritual Awakening (New York: Simon & Schuster, 2012), Kindle edition.

84 "The Lamp and the Key," The Outrageous Wisdom of Nasruddin, accessed May 22, 2019, www.nasruddin.org/pages/storylist. html#lampandkey. I first learned about Mullah Nasruddin listening to lectures by OSHO Rajneesh. Nasruddin, born in present-day Turkey, is considered a populist philosopher, Sufi, and wise man. He is remembered for his amusing stories and anecdotes. This version is my own retelling of a well-known Nasruddin tale to illustrate the comical allegory to depict the biases inherent in many types of scientific research.

(9) "To thine own self be true."

85 Joshua Knobe, "Finding the Mind in the Body," in *Future Science: Essays from the Leading Edge,* ed. Max Brockman (New York: Knopf Doubleday, 2011), Kindle edition.

86 Knobe, "Finding the Mind in the Body."

87 Knobe, "Finding the Mind in the Body."

88 Bryce Huebner, "Commonsense Concepts of Phenomenal Consciousness: Does Anyone Care about Functional Zombies?" *Phenomenology and the Cognitive Sciences* 9, no. 1 (2010): 133–55.

89 Richard Conn Henry, "The Mental Universe," *Nature* 436, no. 7047 (2005): 29.

(10) "Your unconscious mind is a powerhouse."

90 M. Zimmerman, "Neurophysiology of Sensory Systems," in *Fundamentals of Sensory Physiology,* ed. Robert F. Schmidt (Berlin: Springer-Verlag, 1986), 68–116.

91 *Encyclopaedia Britannica,* "Applications of Information Theory:

Physiology" (June 16, 2017), accessed January 25, 2019, https://www.britannica.com/science/information-theory/ Physiology.

92 Tor Nørretranders, *The User Illusion: Cutting Consciousness Down to Size* (London: Penguin, 1999), 277–94.

93 *Encyclopaedia Britannica,* "Applications of Information Theory: Physiology" (June 16, 2017), accessed January 25, 2019, https://www.britannica.com/science/information-theory/ Physiology.

94 Malcolm Gladwell, *Blink: The Power of Thinking Without Thinking* (New York: Little, Brown, 2014), Introduction: The Statue That Didn't Look Right, Kindle edition.

(11) "Consciousness is a continuum of levels."

95 E. F. Schumacher, *A Guide for the Perplexed,* reissued ed. (New York: Harper Perrenial, 2015).

96 Geoffrey Hartman, "Beyond Formalism," *Modern Language Notes* 81, no. 5 (1966): 542–56.

97 John Diamond, *Your Body Doesn't Lie: How to Increase Your Life Energy through Behavioral Kinesiology* (New York: Warner Books, 1983).

98 Dr. Edward Wagner (chiropractor) in discussion with the author, Pacific Palisades, CA, August 2017 and July 2018; Dr. Steven Tonsager (acupuncturist) in discussion with the author, Scottsdale, AZ, February 2019.

99 Robert Frost, *Applied Kinesiology: A Training Manual and Reference Book of Basic Principles and Practices* (Berkeley, CA: North Atlantic Books, 2013), Chapter 3: The Muscle Test. Theory, Procedure, and Interpretation of Muscle Testing,

Kindle edition.

100 David R. Hawkins, *Power vs. Force: The Hidden Determinants of Human Behavior* (Carlsbad, CA: Hay House, 2013), Kindle edition.

(12) "Intention is a process of creation. But first, you have to clear out your crap."

101 Josh Bartok and Chögyam Trungpa Rinpoche, "Searching for the Ox: The Path to Enlightenment in 10 Pictures," *Lions Roar,* March 4, 2015, accessed June 11, 2019, https://www.lionsroar.com/searching-for-the-ox-the-path-to-enlightenment-in-10-pictures/

102 Steven Pressfield, *Turning Pro: Tap Your Inner Power and Create Your Life's Work* (New York, NY: Black Irish Entertainment, 2012), Foreword, Kindle edition.

(13) "We have to go beyond spacetime when we consider consciousness."

103 Vimala Thakar, *Insights into the Bhagavad Gita* (Delhi: Motilal Banarsidass, 2005), 24–25.

104 Stephen Hawking, *A Brief History of Time* (New York: Bantam Books, 2017), Kindle edition.

105 Carlo Rovelli, *The Order of Time,* trans. Erica Segre and Simon Carnell (New York: Penguin, 2018), Chapter 3: Dynamics as Relations, Kindle edition.

106 Rovelli, *The Order of Time,* Chapter 6: The World Is Made Up of Events, Not Things.

107 Cham and Whiteson, *We Have No Idea,* Chapter 7: What Is Space?

108 Franklin Merrell-Wolff, *Pathways through to Space: A*

Personal Record of Transformation in Consciousness (New York: Julian Press, 1973), 241.

(14) "There must be a mathematical formalism between intention and experiment that can be directly tested and quantified."

109 Theodore Melfi, dir., *Hidden Figures* (2017; Beverly Hills, CA: Twentieth Century Fox Home Entertainment, 2017).

110 *Encyclopedia Britannica,* "Differential Equation," accessed April 20, 2019, https://www.britannica.com/science/differential-equation.

111 Schumacher, *A Guide for the Perplexed,* 50.

112 Gingerich, *God's Planet,* Chapter 1: Was Copernicus Right?

BRIDGE PILLAR 3: Of the Mighty Second Law of Thermodynamics, Entropy, And Information

113 Dupre, *Bridges*: Introductory interview, Kindle edition.

114 C. P. Snow, *The Two Cultures and the Scientific Revolution* (Mansfield Center, CT: Martino, 2013), 16.

115 Franco Nori, "Statistical Mechanics and Thermodynamics," *Physics* 406 (Fall 1998), accessed March 14, 2019, http://www-personal.umich.edu/~nori/course/physics_406_quotes.html.

116 William A. Tiller, in Itzhak Bentov, *Stalking the Wild Pendulum: On the Mechanics of Consciousness* (Rochester, VT: Destiny Books, 1988), Preface, Kindle edition.

(15) "Learn thermodynamics. The terms of the second law hold the keys to understanding nature."

117 Hendrick C. Van Ness, *Understanding Thermodynamics* (New

York: McGraw-Hill, 1969), Chapter 1, Kindle edition.

118 Rovelli, *The Order of Time,* Chapter 2, Kindle edition.

(16) "Boltzmann bridged the macroscopic world you see and observe with the microscopic world of atoms."

119 Bill Green, *Boltzmann's Tomb: Travels in Search of Science* (New York: Bellevue Literary Press, 2011), Book Section: Vienna, Kindle edition.

120 Green, Boltzmann's Tomb.

121 Engelbert Broda, *Ludwig Boltzmann: Man, Physicist, Philosopher* (Woodbridge, CT: Ox Bow Press, 1983).

122 Broda, Ludwig Boltzmann, 14.

123 Jean Perrin, *Atoms,* trans. D. L. Hammick (Woodbridge, CT: Ox Bow Press, 1990), Kindle edition.

(17) "Thermodynamics is essential to biology."

124 Axel Kleidon, "Life, Hierarchy, and the Thermodynamic Machinery of Planet Earth," *Physics of Life Reviews* 7, no. 4 (2010): 424–60.

125 Harold J. Morowitz, *Mayonnaise and the Origin of Life: Thoughts of Minds and Molecules* (Woodbridge, CT: Ox Bow Press, 1991).

126 Thomas, *Lives of a Cell: Notes of a Biology Watcher,* Book Section: Lives of a Cell, Kindle edition.

127 Harold J. Morowitz, *Energy Flow in Biology* (Woodbridge, CT: Ox Box Press, 1979).

(18) "People say that life violates the second law of thermodynamics. this is not the case; we know of nothing in the universe that violates that law."

128 Allison Eck, "How Do You Say 'Life' in Physics? A New Theory Sheds Light on the Emergence of Life's Complexity," *Nautilus* (March 17, 2016), accessed April 25, 2019, http://nautil.us/issue/34/adaptation/how-do-you-say-life-in-physics.

129 Noble Media, *The Nobel Prize in Chemistry 1977,* awarded to Ilya Prigogine "for his contributions to non-equilibrium thermodynamics, particularly the theory of dissipative structures, 1977, accessed April 12, 2019, https://www.nobelprize.org/prizes/chemistry/1977/summary/.

130 Gavin E. Crooks, "Beyond Boltzmann-Gibbs Statistics: Maximum Entropy Hyperensembles Out of Equilibrium," *Physical Review. E, Statistical, Nonlinear, and Soft Matter Physics* 75 no. 4, part 1 (2007): 41119.

131 Jeremy England, "Dissipative Adaptation in Driven Self-Assembly," *Nature Nanotechnology* 10, no. 11 (2015): 919; Natalie Wolchover, "A New Physics Theory of Life," *Quanta Magazine,* January 22, 2014, accessed June 25, 2019, https://www.quantamagazine.org/a-new-thermodynamics-theory-of-the-origin-of-life-20140122/ (Simons Foundation: 2014).

132 Brig Klyce, "The Second Law of Thermodynamics," *Cosmic Ancestry,* n.d., accessed April 4, 2019, https://www.panspermia.org/seconlaw.htm#whatsnew.

(19) "The most fundamental aspect of the universe and reality is information. It's more fundamental than matter or energy. Information is the gateway and bridge to understanding ourselves."

133 Harold J. Morowitz, *Entropy for Biologists: An Introduction to Thermodynamics* (New York: Academic Press, 1973), 69.

134 César Hidalgo, *Why Information Grows: The Evolution of*

Order, from Atoms to Economies (New York: Basic Books, 2016), Chapter 2, Kindle edition.

135 C. E. Shannon, "A Mathematical Theory of Communication," *The Bell System Technical Journal* 27, no. 3 (1948): 379–423.

136 M. Mitchell Waldrop, "Claude Shannon: Reluctant Father of the Digital Age," *MIT Technology Review* (July 1, 2001), accessed April 3, 2019, https://www.technologyreview.com/s/401112/claude-shannon-reluctant-father-of-the-digital-age/.

(20) "Information is related to entropy."

137 Morowitz, *Entropy for Biologists,* 108.

138 Tor Nørretranders, *The User Illusion, Cutting Consciousness Down to Size* (London: Penguin, 1999), 23.

139 Léon Brillouin, *Science and Information Theory* (Mineola, NY: Dover, 2013).

140 Morowitz, *Energy Flow in Biology,* 127.

141 Morowitz, *Entropy for Biologists,* 108.

142 Morowitz, *Entropy for Biologists,* 111.

(21) "Entropy and information are crucial to biology."

143 Erwin Schrödinger, *What Is Life?* (Cambridge, UK: Cambridge University Press, 2017), Chapter 6, Kindle edition.

144 Vlatko Vedral, *Decoding Reality: The Universe as Quantum Information* (Oxford, UK: Oxford University Press, 2018), Chapter 5, Kindle edition.

145 Vedral, *Decoding Reality,* Chapter 5, Kindle edition.

BRIDGE PILLAR 4: Four Target Experiments That Bridge Human Intention to Physical Reality in the Laboratory

146 Dupre, *Bridges,* Foreword, Kindle edition.

147 William A. Tiller (physicist) in discussion with the author, Scottsdale, AZ, July 2015.

(22) "Intention is a process of creation."

148 Loren Eiseley, "Water," BrainyQuote.com, accessed March 15, 2019, https://www.brainyquote.com/quotes/loren_eiseley_140840.

149 Roy Rustum, William A. Tiller, Iris Bell, and M. Richard Hoover, "The Structure of Liquid Water; Novel Insights from Materials Research; Potential Relevance to Homeopathy," *Materials Research Innovations* 9, no. 4 (2005): 577–608.

150 "Self-Ionization of Water," *Wikipedia,* accessed April 23, 2019, https://en.wikipedia.org/wiki/Self-ionization_of_water.

151 Rustum et al., "The Structure of Liquid Water," 578.

(23) "We were assisted by the Unseen."

152 William A. Tiller in discussion with the author, Scottsdale, AZ, May 2012.

153 William A. Tiller, Walter E. Dibble, and Michael J. Kohane, "Towards Objectifying Intention via Electronic Devices," *Subtle Energies and Energy Medicine* 8, no. 2 (1999): 103–23; William A. Tiller, Michael J. Kohane, and Walter E. Dibble, "Can an Aspect of Consciousness Be Imprinted into an Electronic Device?" *Integrative Physiological and Behavioral Science* 35, no. 2 (2000): 142–63.

154 Jordan B. Peterson, *12 Rules for Life: An Antidote to Chaos* (Toronto: Random House Canada, 2018), Coda, Kindle edition.

155 William A. Tiller and W. E. Dibble, *White Paper I: A Brief Introduction to Intention-Host Device Research* (Payson, AZ:

William A. Tiller Institute, 2009).

156 Biography.com (June 24, 2015). "James C. Maxwell Biography," accessed April 3, 2019, https://www.biography.com/people/james-c-maxwell-9403463.

(24) "We lost our controls."

157 Richard Hammerschlag et al., "Biofield Research: A Roundtable Discussion of Scientific and Methodological Issues," *Journal of Alternative and Complementary Medicine* 18, no. 12 (2012): 1081–86.

158 Hammerschlag et al., "Biofield Research," 1083.

159 Walter E. Dibble Jr. and William A. Tiller, "Measurement Controls in Anomalies Research," *Journal of Scientific Exploration* 25, no. 2 (2011).

160 Michael J. Kohane and William A. Tiller, "On Enhancing Nicotinamide Adenine Dinucleotide (NAD) Activity in Living Systems," *Subtle Energies and Energy Medicine* 12, no. 3 (2001): 157–81; Dibble and Tiller, "Measurement Controls in Anomalies Research."

161 Kohane and Tiller. "On Enhancing Nicotinamide Adenine Dinucleotide (NAD) Activity in Living Systems," 158–60.

(25) "We can affect materials like water with purely our intention."

162 Walter E. Dibble and William A. Tiller, "Electronic Device-Mediated pH Changes in Water," *Journal of Scientific Exploration* 13, no. 2 (1999): 155–76.

163 Dibble and Tiller, "Electronic Device-Mediated pH Changes in Water," 156.

164 Konstantin Kakaes, *The Pioneer Detectives. Did a Distant Spacecraft Prove Einstein and Newton Wrong?* (The

Millions Online Magazine, 2013), https://themillions.com/original-books/the-pioneer-detectives.

(26) "Intention can enhance biological enzyme function."

165 Ross Firestone, *An Introduction to Enzyme Kinetics*. Khan Academy, Audio-visual on-line academy. Accessed April 23, 2019, https://www.khanacademy.org/test-prep/mcat/biomolecules/enzyme-kinetics/v/an-introduction-to-enzyme-kinetics.

166 Michael J. Kohane and William A. Tiller, "Anomalous Environmental Influences on In Vitro Enzyme Studies. Part 1: Some Faraday Cage and Multiple Vessel Effects," *Subtle Energies and Energy Medicine* 11, no. 1 (2000): 75–97.

167 Michael J. Kohane and William A. Tiller, "Anomalous Environmental Influences on In Vitro Enzyme Studies. Part 2: Some Electronic Device Effects," *Subtle Energies and Energy Medicine* 11, no. 2 (2000): 99–122.

168 Kohane and Tiller, "Anomalous Environmental Influences on In Vitro Enzyme Studies. Part 2," 111.

(27) "The happy fruit flies."

169 Barbara H. Jennings, "*Drosophila*—A Versatile Model in Biology and Medicine," *Materials Today* 14, no. 5 (2011): 190–95.

170 Michael J. Kohane and William A. Tiller, "Energy, Fitness, and Information-Augmented EM Fields in *Drosophila melanogaster*," *Journal of Scientific Exploration* 14, no. 2 (2000): 217–31.

171 Kohane and Tiller, "Energy, Fitness and Information-Augmented EM Fields in Drosophila melanogaster."

172 Kohane and Tiller, "On Enhancing Nicotinamide Adenine

Dinucleotide (NAD) Activity in Living Systems," 157–81.

(28) "Objects can have 'intelligence.'"

173 William A. Tiller (physicist) in discussion with the author, Scottsdale, AZ, November 2014.

174 Tiller, Kohane, and Dibble, "Can an Aspect of Consciousness Be Imprinted into an Electronic Device?" 142–62; discussion 163.

175 Lyall Watson, *The Nature of Things: The Secret Life of Inanimate Objects* (Rochester, VT: Destiny Books, 1992).

176 Jamie Uys, dir., *The Gods Must Be Crazy* (2004; Culver City, CA: Columbia TriStar Home Entertainment, 1980).

177 Joanna Stern, "We Were Promised Mind-Blowing Personal Tech. What's the Hold-Up?" *Wall Street Journal*, May 3, 2018.

BRIDGE PILLAR 5: Of Physical Space and Dual Realities: Beyond the Speed of Light

178 David McCullough, *The Great Bridge: The Epic Story of the Building of the Brooklyn Bridge* (New York: Simon & Schuster, 2012), Epigraph, Kindle edition.

179 Franklin Merrell-Wolff, *Pathways through to Space*, 241.

180 Mary Strong, *Letters of the Scattered Brotherhood* (San Francisco: Harper and Row, 1991), 104.

181 William A. Teller (physicist) in discussion with the author, Scottsdale, AZ, November 2015.

(29) "Physical space is malleable to human intention."

182 William A. Tiller and Walter E. Dibble Jr., "New Experimental Data Revealing an Unexpected Dimension to Materials

Science and Engineering," *Materials Research Innovations* 5, no. 1 (2001): 21–34.

183 Walter E. Dibble Jr. (physicist) in discussion with the author, Payson, AZ, September 2015. The Payson labs are now closed at the time of this writing.

184 Ronald N. Bracewell, "The Fourier Transform," *Scientific American* 260, no. 6 (1989): 86–95; "Fourier Transform," *Wikipedia,* accessed January 18, 2019, https://en.wikipedia.org/wiki/Fourier_transform.

185 Tiller and Dibble, "New Experimental Data Revealing an Unexpected Dimension to Materials Science and Engineering," 21–34.

186 Eberhard Bodenschatz, Werner Pesch, and Guenter Ahlers, "Recent Developments in Rayleigh-Bénard Convection," *Annual Review of Fluid Mechanics* 32, no. 1 (2000): 709–78.

(30) "Paul Dirac coined the term 'empty space.'"

187 Graham Farmelo, *The Strangest Man: The Hidden Life of Paul Dirac,* Quantum Genius (London: Faber, 2010).

188 Frank Wilczek, "A Piece of Magic: The Dirac Equation," *It Must Be Beautiful: Great Equations of Modern Science,* ed. Graham Farmelo (London: Granta, 2003), 132–60.

189 Helge Kragh, *Simply Dirac* (New York: Simply Charly, 2016), Book Section: Anti-Worlds, Kindle edition.

190 CERN, "09 September 1932: Carl Anderson Discovers the Positron," CERN website, accessed February 12, 2019, https://timeline.web.cern.ch/events/carl-anderson-discovers-the-positron.

191 Lederman and T. Hill, Symmetry and the Beautiful Universe,

Chapter 10, Kindle edition.

192 Franklin Merrell-Wolff, *Pathways through to Space,* 158.

193 Paul A. M. Dirac, "Quantised Singularities in the Electromagnetic field," *J Proc. Royal Society.* A 133, no. 821 (1931): 60–72; Paul A. M. Dirac, "The Theory of Magnetic Poles," *Physical Review* 74, no. 7 (1948): 817.

(31) "Space conditioning has a signature with magnetic monopole effects."

194 Tiller and Dibble, "New Experimental Data Revealing an Unexpected Dimension to Materials Science and Engineering," 28.

195 William A. Tiller, Walter E. Dibble Jr., and Michael Kohane, *Conscious Acts of Creation: The Emergence of a New Physics* (Walnut Creek, CA: Pavior, 2001), 173.

(32) "A conditioned space means raising the symmetry of the physical vacuum's electromagnetic state."

196 Hermann Weyl, Symmetry, *Princeton Science Library* reprinted (Princeton, NJ: Princeton University Press, 2016).

197 Gerard 't Hooft, "Gauge Theories of the Forces between Elementary Particles," *Scientific American* 242, no. 6 (June 1980): 104–41.

198 Ian Stewart, *Why Beauty Is Truth: The History of Symmetry* (New York: Basic Books, 2008), 231.

199 Christine Sutton, "Hidden Symmetry: The Yang–Mills Equation," *It Must Be Beautiful: Great Equations of Modern Science,* ed. Graham Farmelo (London: Granta, 2003), 231–52.

200 Sutton, "Hidden Symmetry: The Yang–Mills Equation," 235.

201 Lederman and Hill, *Symmetry and the Beautiful Universe,* Notes, Kindle edition.

202 *Encyclopaedia Britannica,* "Gauge Theory," accessed April 3, 2019, https://www.britannica.com/science/gauge-theory.

203 Dave Goldberg, *The Universe in the Rearview Mirror: How Hidden Symmetries Shape Reality* (New York: Plume, 2014), Kindle edition.

(33) "Space conditioning requires a new type of reference frame than just space-time for viewing nature."

204 William A. Tiller, "Towards a Predictive Model of Subtle Domain Connections to the Physical Domain Aspect of Reality: The Origins of Wave-Particle Duality, Electric-Magnetic Monopoles and the Mirror Principle," *Journal of Scientific Exploration* 13, no. 1 (1999): 41–67.

205 Encyclopaedia Britannica, "De Broglie Wave," accessed February 15, 2019, https://www.britannica.com/science/de-Broglie-wave.

206 Sal Khan, "Intro to Inverse Functions" In *Math, Algebra II, Functions, Introduction to Inverse Functions,* Khan Academy, accessed March 15, 2019. https://www. khanacademy.org/math/algebra2/manipulating-functions/ introduction-to-inverses-of-functions/v/introduction-to-function-inverses.

207 Cham and Whiteson, *We Have No Idea,* Chapter 3: What Is Dark Energy?

(34) "There is higher thermodynamic free energy available in conditioned space."

208 *Encyclopaedia Britannica,* "Electron volt," accessed May 21,

2019, https://www.britannica.com/science/electron-volt.

209 William A. Tiller and Walter Dibble Jr., "Expanding Thermodynamic Perspective for Materials in SU (2) EM Gauge Symmetry State Space: Part 2–Magnetoelectrochemical Potential Energy Detector," *Materials Research Innovations* 12, no. 3 (2008): 107–113.

210 William A. Tiller, "Electromagnetism versus Bioelectromagnetism," in *Bioelectromagnetic and Subtle Energy Medicine,* 2nd edn., ed. Paul. J. Rosch (Boca Raton, FL: CRC Press, 2015), Chapter 7, Kindle edition.

(35) "There is another communication channel in nature. The R-space is the medium whereby information is transferred. It is information entanglement."

211 Tiller, *Psychoenergetic Science,* 98–99.

212 William A. Tiller et al., "Toward General Experimentation and Discovery in Conditioned Laboratory Spaces: Part IV. Macroscopic Information Entanglement between Sites Approximately 6000 Miles Apart," *Journal of Alternative and Complementary Medicine* 11, no. 6 (2005): 973–76.

213 Watson, *The Nature of Things,* 47.

(36) "I postulate a new particle, deltron, that connects direct-space with reciprocal space."

214 Tiller, *Psychoenergetic Science,* 128–29.

(37) "Humans create field effects."

215 William A. Tiller, *Psychoenergetic Science: A Second Copernican-Scale Revolution* (Lecture series, University of Denver, Denver, CO: 2007). Five DVD set. Available from

www.tiller.org.

216 Steven Pressfield, *The War of Art: Break through the Blocks and Win Your Inner Creative Battles* (New York: Black Irish Entertainment, 2012), Foreword, Kindle edition.

(38) "The term 'zero-point energy' is misunderstood by the general public to mean something to do with consciousness."

217 "Polar Vortex Triggers Coldest Arctic Outbreak in at Least Two Decades in Parts of the Midwest," The Weather Channel, accessed January 31, 2019, https://weather.com/forecast/national/news/2019-01-28-polar-vortex-midwest-arctic-air-coldest-two-decades.
I was in Bemidji, Minnesota during the historic polar vortex. My rental car froze and became like a huge hockey puck. With a wind chill of minus 65 degrees centigrade, the temperature in the deep freezer section of a refrigerator was warmer than the outdoors! The polar temperatures gave me a new perspective of thermal motion and heat. Believe me, my intention was to get in and stay in a warm room.

218 "MIT Team Achieves Coldest Temperature Ever," *MIT News*, September 11, 2003, accessed January 16, 2019, http://news.mit.edu/2003/cooling.

219 Philip Yam, "Exploiting Zero-Point Energy," *Scientific American* 277, no. 6 (1997): 82–85.

220 *The Nobel Prize in Physics 1978*. 1978, accessed April 23, 2019, https://www.nobelprize.org/prizes/physics/1978/summary/.

221 Tom Shachtman, "The Coldest Place in the Universe," *Smithsonian Magazine,* January 2008, accessed April 3, 2019, https://www.smithsonianmag.com/science-nature/the-

coldest-place-in-the-universe-8121922/.

BRIDGE PILLAR 6: Subtle Energy and Information Medicine for The Twenty-First Century: Subluminal and Superluminal Bridge Together.

222 Franklin Merrell-Wolff, *Pathways through to Space*, 25.

223 William A. Tiller (physicist) in discussion with the author, Scottsdale, AZ, October 2014.

(39) "The acupuncture system is the energy pump in the human body."

224 William A. Tiller (physicist) in discussion with the author, Scottsdale, AZ, June 2015.

225 R. C. Niemtzow, "Acupuncture and Magnets: Is There a Clinical Role?" *Medical Acupuncture* 29, no. 5 (2017): 255–56.

226 "Dr. Issac Goiz Durán Biography," Goiz Biomagnetism, 2018, accessed March 17, 2019, http://isaacgoiz.com/english.html

227 Bryan L. Frank, "Biomagnetic Pair Therapy and Typhoid Fever: A Pilot Study," *Medical Acupuncture* 29, no. 5 (2017): 308–12.

228 Robert Frost, *The Muscle Test: Theory, Procedure, and Interpretation of Muscle Testing in Applied Kinesiology* (Berkeley, CA: North Atlantic Books, 2013), Chapter 3: The Muscle Test, Kindle edition.

229 Paul J. Rosch, *Bioelectromagnetic and Subtle Energy Medicine,* 2nd edn. (Boca Raton, FL: CRC Press, 2015), Chapter 1, Kindle edition.

230 Niemtzow, "Acupuncture and Magnets, 255–56.

231 William A. Tiller, "White Paper XV: Preventive Medicine/Self-Healing via One's Personal Biofield Pumping and Balancing" (Payson, AZ: William A. Tiller Institute, n.d.).

232 William A. Tiller, Elmer E. Green, Peter A. Parks, and Stacy
     Anderson, "Towards Explaining Anomalously Large
     Body Voltage Surges on Exceptional Subjects. Part I:
     The Electrostatic Approximation," *Journal of Scientific
     Exploration* 9, no. 3 (1995): 331–50.
233 William A. Tiller, "The Real World of Modern Science,
     Medicine, and Qigong," *Bulletin of Science, Technology and
     Society* 22, no. 5 (2002): 352–61.

(40) "My research has led me to develop personal practices for subtle energy balancing and pumping."

234 Leslie Patten and Terry Patten, *Biocircuits: Amazing New
     Tools for Energy Health* (Tiburon, CA: H. J. Kramer, 1989),
     24–25.
235 Leon Ernest Eeman, *Cooperative Healing: The Curative
     Properties of Human Radiations* (Frederick Muller, 1947).
236 William A. Tiller, "White Paper XV: Preventive Medicine."
237 Patton and Patton, Biocircuits, 29–31.

(41) "Healing spaces can be created where people feel safe and well."

238 C. W. Smith, "CAM in Camera," *Journal of Alternative and
     Complementary Medicine* 13, no. 1 (2007): 3–4.
239 William A. Tiller and Walter E. Dibble, "Toward General
     Experimentation and Discovery in Conditioned Laboratory
     and Complementary and Alternative Medicine Spaces:
     Part V. Data on 10 Different Sites Using a Robust New Type
     of Subtle Energy Detector," *Journal of Alternative and
     Complementary Medicine* 13, no. 1 (2007): 133–49.
240 Grazyna A. Pajunen, Marguerite J. Purnell, Walter E. Dibble

Jr, and William A. Tiller, "Altering the Acid/Alkaline Balance of Water via the Use of an Intention-Host Device," *Journal of Alternative and Complementary Medicine* 15, no. 9 (2009): 963–68.

241 Alex Hankey, "The Thermodynamics of Healing, Health, and Love," *Journal of Alternative and Complementary Medicine* 13, no. 1 (2007): 5–8.

(42) "Information medicine is the way of the future."

242 J. Baio et al., "Prevalence of Autism Spectrum Disorder among Children Aged 8 Years—Autism and Developmental Disabilities Monitoring Network, 11 Sites, United States, 2014," *MMWR Surveillance Summaries: Morbidity and Mortality Weekly Report* 67, no. 6 (2018): 1–23.

243 Suzy Miller, *Awesomism! A New Way to Understand the Diagnosis of Autism* (n.p.: iUniverse, 2008).

244 Autism Research Institute, accessed May 19, 2019, https://www.autism.org/atec; I. Magiati et al., "Is the Autism Treatment Evaluation Checklist a Useful Tool for Monitoring Progress in Children with Autism Spectrum Disorders?" *Intellectual Disabilities,* 55, no. 3 (2011): 302–12.

245 Gregory Fandel (personal assistant to William A. Tiller) in discussion with the author, Scottsdale, AZ, October 2018.

246 William A. Tiller, S. Miller, C. R. Reed, and J. Yotopoulos, "White Paper XXX, The Globally Broadcast Autism Intention Experiment: Part I, at the Four-Month Stage of a Twelve-Month Program" (Payson, AZ: Tiller Institute, 2013).

247 William A. Tiller, S. Miller, C.R. Reed, F. Tang, N. Manek, and W.E. Dibble, "White Paper XXXI, The Globally Broadcast

Autism Intention Experiment: Part II. Some ATEC Trends and Statistical Data for a Twelve-month Program" (Payson, AZ: Tiller Institute, 2014), 5.

248 Tiller, Miller, Reed, and Yotopoulos, "White Paper XXX, The Globally Broadcast Autism Intention Experiment, Part I," 14."

249 Suzy Miller, C. Reed, F. Tang, N. J. Manek, and W. A. Tiller, *Impact of Broadcast Intention on Autism Spectrum Behaviors, in International Research Congress on Integrative Medicine and Health (IRCIMH)* (Miami, FL: 2014), Conference paper.

250 D. Harner, "Proposal for a Non-Distance-Time Framework for the Healing Arts" (PhD diss., California Institute of Human Science, 2015).

251 Galileo Galilei, 1564–1642, and Giovanni Gentile, *Frammenti E Lettere* (Livorno, Italy: R. Giusti, 1917).

(43) "Many people are deficient in self-acceptance."

252 Vivek Murthy, "Work and the Loneliness Epidemic: Reducing Isolation at Work Is Good for Business," *Harvard Business Review,* September, 2017.

253 Merrit Kennedy, "U.K. Now Has a Minister for Loneliness," *The Two-Way, NPR,* accessed January 17, 2018, https://www.npr.org/sections/thetwo-way/2018/01/17/578645954/u-k-now-has-a-minister-for-loneliness.

254 William A. Tiller, *Science and Human Transformation: Subtle Energies, Intentionality, and Consciousness* (Walnut Creek, CA: Pavior, 1997), 216.

255 Kristin D. Neff, "The Development and Validation of a Scale to Measure Self-Compassion," *Self and Identity* 2, no. 3 (2003):

223–50.

256 Richard W. Robins, Holly M. Hendin, and Kali H. Trzesniewski, "Measuring Global Self-Esteem: Construct Validation of a Single-Item Measure and the Rosenberg Self-Esteem Scale," *Personality and Social Psychology Bulletin* 27, no. 2 (2001): 151–61.

257 Gabriele T. Hilberg, William A. Tiller, "Self-Criticism to Self-Compassion: A Proof of Concept Study Utilizing Intention Broadcast," *Institute of Noetic Science (IONS).* (Chicago, IL: 2015, IONS), Conference paper.

258 Gabriele Hilberg (psychologist) in discussion with the author via email, December 30, 2018.

259 David R. Hawkins, *Letting Go: The Pathway of Surrender* (Carlsbad, CA: Hay House, 2013).

(44) "Information medicine is personalized medicine."

260 Nisha J. Manek and William A. Tiller, "Information Medicine as Delivered by Intention Host Devices: A Case Report," *International Research Congress on Integrative Medicine and Health.* (2014, IRCIMH: Miami, FL), Conference paper.

261 S. Garrett, T. Jenkinson, L. G. Kennedy, H. Whitelock, P. Gaisford, and A. Calin, "A New Approach to Defining Disease Status in Ankylosing spondylitis: The Bath Ankylosing Spondylitis Disease Activity Index," J Rheumatol 21(12, 1994): 2286–291, accessed March 16, 2019, http://www.basdai.com/.

262 William A. Tiller (physicist), in discussion with the author, Scottsdale, AZ, November 2015.

(45) "Consciousness beats lifestyle."

263 Hawkins, *Power vs. Force,* Chapter 20, Kindle edition.

BRIDGE PILLAR 7: Of Thermodynamics, Love, And Becoming *Homo spiritus.*

264 Merrell-Wolff, *Pathways through to Space,* 105.

265 Jimmy Soni and Rob Goodman, *A Mind at Play: How Claude Shannon Invented the Information Age* (New York: Simon &Schuster, 2018), Kindle edition.

266 William Tiller (physicist), in discussion with the author, Scottsdale, AZ, November 2015. Tiller's marvelous aphorism is striking to me. His lab, his intention, his protocol are no different than a Spiritual protocol to seek the Truth.

(46) "It is not a traditional force that radiates from the relics of the historical Buddha."

267 Nisha J. Manek, "Symmetry States of the Physical Space: An Expanded Reference Frame for Understanding Human Consciousness," *Journal of Alternative and Complementary Medicine* 18, no. 1 (2012): 83–92.

268 Manek, "Symmetry States of the Physical Space," 85.

269 Watson, *The Nature of Things,* 148.

(47) "Thermodynamics of Loving-kindness can be measured."

270 William A. Tiller, Jean E. Tiller, Walter E. Dibble, Raj Manek, and Nisha J. Manek, "The Buddha Relics and Evidence of Physical Space Conditioning with Unimprinted Intention Host Devices," *Journal of Alternative and Complementary Medicine* 18, no. 4 (2012): 379–81.

271 William A. Tiller et al., "The Buddha Relics," 380.

(48) "The Buddha relics show us the answer to mankind's age-old question: Does consciousness survive physical death?"
(no notes)

(49) "Nothing is causing anything."
272 "International System of Units Revised in Historic Vote," Bureau International des Poids et Mesures, accessed February 14, 2019, https://www.bipm.org/en/news/full-stories/2018-11-si-overhaul.html.

(50) "We can reach for the stars."
273 Encyclopaedia Britannica, "John Archibald Wheeler," accessed April 4, 2019, https://www.britannica.com/biography/John-Archibald-Wheeler.
274 Tiller, "What Are Subtle Energies," 293–304; Leon M. Lederman and Christopher Hill, *Beyond the God Particle* (Amherst, NY: Prometheus Books, 2013), Chapter 9, Kindle edition.
275 Thakar, *Insights into the Bhagavad Gita,* 168.

(51) "Brighten the corner where you are."
(no notes)

(52) "Mankind is evolving to adepts, masters, and avatars by the tool of intention."
276 "E. F. Schumacher Quotes," AZQuotes, accessed April 4, 2019, https://www.azquotes.com/author/13159-E_F_Schumacher?p=3.
277 Anya Sophia Mann, "Science and Spirituality: The Perfect Union," Quantum Alchemy Radio, July 9, 2014. Available

from, http://AnyaSophiaMann.com.

278 David R. Hawkins, "Seminar on Human Consciousness and Evolution, Sedona Creative Life Center, Sedona, AZ." Hawkins said a version of this statement many times. This version is the author's retelling of his overall theme on human consciousness and evolution.

279 Sermon, Endeavor Academy, Wisconsin Dells, WI, July 2011.

280 Vimala Thakar (spiritual teacher) in discussion with the author at "Shiv-Kuti," Mt. Abu, Rajasthan, India, September 2006.

Afterword

281 Arthritis Foundation, Your Exercise Solution: Tai Chi. The Arthritis Resource Finder is an online resource to help you locate a tai chi class in your area. The Arthritis Foundation also offers a tai chi DVD created especially for people with arthritis. https://www.arthritis.org/living-with-arthritis/exercise/arthritis-friendly/tai-chi.php.

282 The Maitreya Buddha Project is being developed in Kushinagar, India, where Shakyamuni Buddha showed the holy deed of passing away and where the future Buddha Maitreya will take birth. As I see it, the Maitreya Buddha statue broadcasts, that is, radiates Loving-kindness to all sentient beings around Earth. As Lama Thubten Zopa Rinpoche says: "Our main goal is not the Maitreya Buddha statue itself. The main goal is the peace and happiness of all living beings ..." http://mbpkushinagar.org/.

Acknowledgments

283 Fran Grace, The Power of Love: A Transformed Heart Changes

the World (Redlands, CA: Inner Pathway, 2019).

284 California Institute of Human Science: https://www.cihs.edu/.

285 Spring Forest Qigong Center: https://www.springforestqigong.com/.

286 Flowing Rivers Acupuncture, 1694 Commerce Ct., River Falls, WI 54022.

287 Patricia A. Lynch, *Letters to God: Transforming Crisis into Consciousness* (Cottonwood, AZ: Mingus Mountain Publishing, 2018).

288 Joseph Gallenberger, *Inner Vegas: Creating Miracles, Abundances, and Health* (Faber, VA: Rainbow Ridge Books, 2013).

289 Susan E. Flint and Raj Rajkumar, *Artificial Intelligence: The Final Dominion* (n.p.: SuRaj Publications, 2018), Kindle edition.

BIBLIOGRAPHY

23andMeBlog. "Genetic Similarities of Mice and Men." Genetics 1010, 23andMeBlog, April 20, 2012. Accessed January 15, 2019. https://blog.23andme.com/23andme-and-you/genetics-101/genetic-similarities-of-mice-and-men/.

Alexander, Eben. *Into the Afterlife: A Neurosurgeon's Near-Death Experience and Spiritual Awakening.* New York: Simon & Schuster, 2012. Kindle.

Autism Research Institute. Accessed May 19, 2019. https://www.autism.org/atec.

Baio, J., L. Wiggins, D. L. Christensen, M. J. Maenner, J. Daniels, Z. Warren, M. Kurzius-Spencer et al. "Prevalence of Autism Spectrum Disorder among Children Aged 8 Years – Autism and Developmental Disabilities Monitoring Network, 11 Sites, United States, 2014." *MMWR Surveillance Summaries: Morbidity and Mortality Weekly Report* 67, no. 6 (2018): 1–23.

Bartok, Josh, and Chögyam Trungpa Rinpoche. "Searching for the Ox: The Path to Enlightenment in 10 Pictures." Lion's Roar, March 4, 2015. Accessed June 11, 2019. www.lionsroar.com/searching-for-the-ox-the-path-to-enlightenment-in-10-pictures/.

Bentov, Itzhak. *Stalking the Wild Pendulum: On the Mechanics of Consciousness.* Rochester, VT: Destiny Books, 1988. Kindle.

Bhagavatpada, Adishankara. "Shivanandalahari." English Translation. Accessed May 21, 2019. https://shaivam.org/scripture/English-Translation/1433/shivanandalahari-by-adishankara-bhagavatpada-english-translation.

Biography.com. "James C. Maxwell Biography." June 24, 2015. Accessed April 3, 2019. www.biography.com/people/james-c-maxwell-9403463.

Bodenschatz, Eberhard, Werner Pesch, and Guenter Ahlers. "Recent Developments in Rayleigh-Bénard Convection." *Annual Review of Fluid Mechanics* 32, no. 1 (2000): 709–78.

Bracewell, Ronald N. "The Fourier Transform." *Scientific American* 260, no. 6 (1989): 86–95.

Brillouin, Leon. *Science and Information Theory.* Mineola, NY: Dover, 2013.

Broda, Engelbert. *Ludwig Boltzmann: Man, Physicist, Philosopher.* Woodbridge, CT: Ox Bow Press, 1983.

Buchanan, Lyn. *The Seventh Sense: The Secrets of Remote Viewing as Told by a "Psychic Spy" for the U.S. Military.* New York: Paraview Pocket, 2003. Kindle.

Center, C., M. Davis, T. Detre, D. E. Ford, W. Hansbrough, H. Hendin, J. Laszlo et al. "Confronting Depression and Suicide in Physicians: A Consensus Statement." *Journal of the American Medical Association* 289, no. 23 (2003): 3161–66.

Central Intelligence Agency. *DOD Psychoenergetics Program,* DoD. 2016.

CERN. "09 September 1932: Carl Anderson Discovers the Positron." Accessed February 12, 2019. https://timeline.web.cern.ch/events/carl-anderson-discovers-the-positron.

CERN. "The Large Hadron Collider." Accessed January 3, 2019. https://home.cern/science/accelerators/large-hadron-collider.

CERN. "Lord Shiva Statue Unveiled." *CERN Bulletin* 27 (2004). Accessed January 30, 2019. https://cds.cern.ch/

record/745737/?ln=en.

Chalmers, David J. "Facing up to the Problem of Consciousness." *Journal of Consciousness Studies* 2, no. 3 (1995): 200–219.

Cham, Jorge, and Daniel Whiteson. *We Have No Idea: A Guide to the Unknown Universe.* New York: Penguin, 2017. Kindle.

Clarke, Tainya C., Lindsey I. Black, Barbara J. Stussman, Patricia M. Barnes, and Richard L. Nahin. "Trends in the Use of Complementary Health Approaches among Adults: United States, 2002–2012." *National Health Statistics Reports,* no. 79 (2015): 1–16.

Crooks, Gavin E. "Beyond Boltzmann-Gibbs Statistics: Maximum Entropy Hyperensembles out of Equilibrium." *Physical Review. E, Statistical, Nonlinear, and Soft Matter Physics* 75, no. 4, part 1 (2007): 041119.

Descartes, René. *Delphi Collected Works of René Descartes.* Location: Delphi Series Seven, Book 25, Delphi Classics. Kindle.

Descartes, René. *Discourse on the Method of Rightly Conducting One's Reason and of Seeking Truth in the Sciences.* Hamburg, Germany: Tredition Classics, 2012. Kindle.

Diamond, John. *Your Body Doesn't Lie: How to Increase Your Life Energy through Behavioral Kinesiology.* New York: Warner Books, 1983.

Dibble Jr., Walter E., and William A. Tiller. "Electronic Device-Mediated pH Changes in Water." *Journal of Scientific Exploration* 13, no. 2 (1999): 155–76.

Dibble Jr., Walter E., and William A. Tiller. "Measurement Controls in Anomalies Research." *Journal of Scientific Exploration* 25, no. 2 (2011): 237–64.

Dirac, P.A.M. "Quantised Singularities in the Electromagnetic

Field." *J Proc. Royal Society.* A 133, no. 821 (1931): 60–72.

Dirac, P.A.M. "The Theory of Magnetic Poles." *Physical Review* 74, no. 7 (1948): 817.

Downing, N. S., N. D. Shah, J. A. Aminawung, A. M. Pease, J. D. Zeitoun, H. M. Krumholz, J. S. Ross. "Postmarket Safety Events among Novel Therapeutics Approved by the US Food and Drug Administration between 2001 and 2010." *Journal of the American Medical Association* 317, no. 18 (2017): 1854–63.

Dupre, Judith. *Bridges: A History of the World's Most Spectacular Spans.* New York: Running Press, 2017. Kindle.

Eck, Allison. "How Do You Say 'Life' in Physics? A New Theory Sheds Light on the Emergence of Life's Complexity." *Nautilus* 34 (July 20, 2017). Accessed March 17, 2019. http://nautil.us/issue/34/adaptation/how-do-you-say-life-in-physics.

Eeman, L. E. *Cooperative Healing: The Curative Properties of Human Radiations.* n.p.: Frederick Muller, 1947.

Eiseley, L., *Water.* BrainyQuote. Accessed March 15, 2019. www.brainyquote.com/quotes/loren_eiseley_140840.

Encyclopaedia Britannica. "Applications of Information Theory: Physiology." Accessed January 25, 2019. www.britannica.com/science/information-theory/Physiology.

Encyclopaedia Britannica. "De Broglie Wave." Accessed February 15, 2019. www.britannica.com/science/de-Broglie-wave.

Encyclopaedia Britannica, "Differential Equation." Accessed April 21, 2019. www.britannica.com/science/differential-equation.

Encyclopaedia Britannica, "Electron volt." Accessed May 21, 2019. www.britannica.com/science/electron-volt.

Encyclopaedia Britannica. "Gauge Theory." Accessed April 3, 2019. www.britannica.com/science/gauge-theory.

Encyclopaedia Britannica. "John Archibald Wheeler." Accessed April 4, 2019. www.britannica.com/biography/John-Archibald-Wheeler.

England, Jeremy. "Dissipative Adaptation in Driven Self-Assembly." *Nature Nanotechnology* 10, no. 11 (2015): 919–923.

Farmelo, Graham. *The Strangest Man: The Hidden Life of Paul Dirac, Quantum Genius.* London: Faber, 2010.

Firestone, Ross. *An Introduction to Enzyme Kinetics.* Khan Academy, Audio-visual on-line academy. Accessed April 23, 2019. www.khanacademy.org/test-prep/mcat/biomolecules/enzyme-kinetics/v/an-introduction-to-enzyme-kinetics.

Flint, Susan E., and Raj Rajkumar. *Artificial Intelligence: The Final Dominion.* n.p.: Suraj Publications, 2018.

"Fourier Transform." *Wikipedia.* Accessed January 18, 2019. https://en.wikipedia.org/wiki/Fourier_transform.

Frank, Bryan L. "Biomagnetic Pair Therapy and Typhoid Fever: A Pilot Study." *Medical Acupuncture* 29, no. 5 (2017): 308–12.

Frost, Robert. *Applied Kinesiology: A Training Manual and Reference Book of Basic Principles and Practices.* Berkeley, CA: North Atlantic Books, 2013. Kindle.

Frost, Robert. *The Muscle Test: Theory, Procedure, and Interpretation of Muscle Testing in Applied Kinesiology.* Berkeley, CA: North Atlantic Books. 2013. Kindle.

Galilei, Galileo, and Giovanni Gentile. *Frammenti E Lettere.* Livorno, Italy: R. Giusti, 1917.

Gallenberger, Joseph. *Inner Vegas: Creating Miracles, Abundances, and Health.* Faber, VA: Rainbow Ridge Books, 2013.

Garrett, S., T. Jenkinson, L. G. Kennedy, H. Whitelock, P. Gaisford, and A. Calin. "A New Approach to Defining Disease Status in Ankylosing Spondylitis: The Bath Ankylosing Spondylitis

Disease Activity Index." *J Rheumatol* 21, no. 12(1994): 2286–91. Accessed March 16, 2019. www.basdai.com.

Gaukroger, Stephen. *Descartes: An Intellectual Biography.* Oxford, UK: Clarendon, 2003.

Gladwell, Malcolm. *Blink: The Power of Thinking Without Thinking.* New York: Little, Brown, 2014. Kindle.

Goiz Biomagnetism. "Dr. Issac Goiz Durán Biography." Accessed March 17, 2019. http://isaacgoiz.com/english.html.

Goldberg, Dave. *The Universe in the Rearview Mirror: How Hidden Symmetries Shape Reality.* New York: Plume, 2014. Kindle.

Graff, D. E., and P. S. Cyrus. *Perceiving the Future News: Evidence for Retrocausation.* In *American Institute of Physics.* AIP Conference Proceedings 1841, 030001 (2017). https://doi.org/10.1063/1.4982772.

Gingerich, Owen. *God's Planet.* Cambridge, MA: Harvard University Press, 2014. Kindle.

Gingerich, Owen. *God's Universe.* Cambridge, MA: Belknap, 2006.

Grace, Fran. *The Power of Love: A Transformed Heart Changes the World.* Redlands, CA: Inner Pathway, 2019.

Green, Bill. *Boltzmann's Tomb: Travels in Search of Science.* New York: Bellevue Literary Press, 2011. Kindle.

Guarneri, Erminia, and Rauni Prittinen King. "Challenges and Opportunities Faced by Biofield Practitioners in *Global Health and Medicine: A White Paper.*" Global Advances in Health and Medicine 4, supplement (2015): 89–96.

Hameroff, Stuart, and Roger Penrose. "Consciousness in the Universe: A Review of the 'Orch OR' Theory." *Physics of Life Reviews* 11, no. 1 (2014): 39–78.

Hammerschlag, Richard, et al. "Biofield Research: A Roundtable

Discussion of Scientific and Methodological Issues." *Journal of Alternative and Complementary Medicine* 18, no. 12 (2012): 1081–86.

Hankey, Alex. "The Thermodynamics of Healing, Health, and Love." *Journal of Alternative and Complementary Medicine* 13, no. 1 (2007): 5–8.

Harner, D. "Proposal for a Non-Distance-Time Framework for the Healing Arts." PhD diss., California Institute of Human Science, 2015.

Hartman, Geoffrey. "Beyond Formalism." *Modern Language Notes* 81, no. 5 (1966): 542–56.

Hawking, Stephen. *A Brief History of Time*. New York: Bantam Books, 2017. Kindle.

Hawkins, David R. *Letting Go: The Pathway of Surrender*. Carlsbad, CA: Hay House, 2013.

Hawkins, David R. *Power vs. Force: The Hidden Determinants of Human Behavior*. Carlsbad, CA: Hay House, 2013. Kindle.

"High Impact Journals: Superfund Research Program." National Institute of Environmental Health Sciences website. Accessed January 24, 2019. https://tools.niehs.nih.gov/srp/publications/highimpactjournals.cfm.

Henry, Richard Conn. "The Mental Universe." *Nature* 436, no. 7047 (2005): 29.

Hidalgo, César. *Why Information Grows: The Evolution of Order, from Atoms to Economies*. New York: Basic Books, 2016. Kindle.

Hilberg, G. T., WA. "Self-Critism to Self-Compassion: A Proof of Concept Study Utilizing Intention Broadcast." *Institute of Noetic Science (IONS)*. Chicago, IL: IONS, 2015.

Huebner, Bryce. "Commonsense Concepts of Phenomenal

Consciousness: Does Anyone *Care* about Functional Zombies?" *Phenomenology and the Cognitive Sciences* 9, no. 1 (2010): 133–55.

"International System of Units Revised in Historic Vote." Bureau International des Poids et Mesures. Accessed February 14, 2019. www.bipm.org/en/news/full-stories/2018-11-si-overhaul.html.

Jahn, Robert G., and Brenda J. Dunne. *Margins of Reality: The Role of Consciousness in the Physical World*. Princeton, NJ: ICRL Press, 2009. Kindle.

Jasanoff, Alan. *The Biological Mind: How Brain, Body, and Environment Collaborate to Make Us Who We Are*. New York: Basic Books, 2018. Kindle edition.

Jennings, Barbara H. "*Drosophila*—A Versatile Model in Biology and Medicine." *Materials Today* 14, no. 5 (2011): 190–95.

Kakaes, Konstantin. *The Pioneer Detectives. Did a Distant Spacecraft Prove Einstein and Newton Wrong?* eBook: The Millions, 2013.

Kemper, Kathi J. *Authentic Healing: A Practical Guide for Caregivers*. Minneapolis, MN: Two Harbors Press, 2016.

Kennedy, Merrit. "U.K. Now Has a Minister for Loneliness." The Two-Way, NPR, January 17, 2018. Accessed January 15, 2019. www.npr.org/sections/thetwo-way/2018/01/17/578645954/u-k-now-has-a-minister-for-loneliness.

Khan Academy. "An Introduction to Enzyme Kinetics." Accessed April 23, 2019. www.khanacademy.org/test-prep/mcat/biomolecules/enzyme-kinetics/v/an-introduction-to-enzyme-kinetics.

Khan Academy. "Nicolaus Copernicus: A Sun-Centered View of the Universe." *How Did Our View of the Universe Change?* Accessed

March 11, 2019. www.khanacademy.org/partner-content/big-history-project/big-bang/how-did-big-bang-change/a/nicolaus-copernicus-bh.

Khan, Sal. "Intro to Inverse Functions," *Math, Algebra II, Functions, Introduction to Inverse Functions.* Khan Academy. Accessed March 15, 2019. www.khanacademy.org/math/algebra2/manipulating-functions/introduction-to-inverses-of-functions/v/introduction-to-function-inverses.

Kleidon, Axel. "Life, Hierarchy, and the Thermodynamic Machinery of Planet Earth." *Physics of Life Reviews* 7, no. 4 (2010): 424–60.

Klyce, Brig. "The Second Law of Thermodynamics." *Cosmic Ancestry,* n.d. Accessed April 4, 2019. www.panspermia.org/seconlaw.htm#whatsnew.

Knobe, Joshua. "Finding the Mind in the Body." *Future Science: Essays from the Cutting Edge,* edited by Max Brockman, 184–96. New York: Vintage, 2011.

Kohane, Michael J., and William A. Tiller. "Anomalous Environmental Influences on *In Vitro* Enzyme Studies. Part 1: Some Faraday Cage and Multiple Vessel Effects." *Subtle Energies and Energy Medicine* 11, no. 1 (2000): 75–97.

Kohane, Michael J., and William A. Tiller. "Anomalous Environmental Influences on *In Vitro* Enzyme Studies. Part 2: Some Electronic Device Effects." *Subtle Energies and Energy Medicine* 11, no. 2 (2000): 99–122.

Kohane, Michael J., and William A. Tiller. "Energy, Fitness, and Information-Augmented EM Fields in *Drosophila melanogaster.*" *Journal of Scientific Exploration* 14, no. 2 (2000): 217–31.

Kohane, Michael J., and William A. Tiller. "On Enhancing

Nicotinamide Adenine Dinucleotide (NAD) Activity in Living Systems." *Subtle Energies and Energy Medicine* 12, no. 3 (2001): 157–81.

Kragh, Helge. *Simply Dirac.* New York: Simply Charly, 2016. Kindle.

Lederman, Leon M., and Christopher Hill. *Beyond the God Particle.* Amherst, NY: Prometheus Books, 2013. Kindle.

Lederman, Leon M., and Christopher T. Hill. *Symmetry and the Beautiful Universe.* Amherst, NY: Prometheus, 2014. Kindle.

Le Fanu, James. *The Rise & Fall of Modern Medicine.* London: Abacus Software, 2014.

Le Fanu, James. *Too Many Pills: How Too Much Medicine Is Endangering Our Health and What We Can Do About It.* New York: Little, Brown, 2018.

Lin, Chunyi, and Gary Rebstock. *Born a Healer.* Eden Prairie, MN: Spring Forest, 2003.

Lynch, Patricia A. *Letters to God: Transforming Crisis into Consciousness.* Cottonwood, AZ: Mingus Mountain Publishing, 2018.

Magiati, I., et al. "Is the Autism Treatment Evaluation Checklist a Useful Tool for Monitoring Progress in Children with Autism Spectrum Disorders?" *Intellectual Disabilities* 55, no. 3 (2011): 302–12.

Manek, N. J. "Symmetry States of the Physical Space: An Expanded Reference Frame for Understanding Human Consciousness." *Journal of Alternative and Complementary Medicine* 18, no. 1 (2012): 83–92.

Manek, N. J., and Chunyi Lin. "Qigong." *Textbook of Complementary and Alternative Medicine.* 2nd ed. Edited by Chun-Su Yuan, Eric J. Bieber, and Brent Bauer, 199–210. Boca

Raton, FL: CRC Press, 2006.

Manek, N. J., and William A. Tiller. "Information Medicine as Delivered by Intention Host Devices: A Case Report." In *International Research Congress on Integrative Medicine and Health*. Miami, FL: IRCIMH, 2014.

Manek, N. J., C. S. Crowson, A. L. Ottenberg, F. A. Curlin, T. J. Kaptchuk, and J. C. Tilburt. "What Rheumatologists in the United States Think of Complementary and Alternative Medicine: Results of a National Survey." *BMC Complementary and Alternative Medicine* 10 (2010): 5.

Mann, Anya Sophia. "Science and Spirituality: The Perfect Union." *Quantum Alchemy Radio,* July 9, 2014. Available from http://AnyaSophiaMann.com.

Maritain, Jacques. *The Dream of Descartes*. Translated by M.L.C. Andison. London: Editions Poetry London, 1946.

Marshall, Barry. "*Helicobacter pylori*–A Nobel Pursuit?" *Canadian Journal of Gastroenterology* 22, no. 11 (2008): 895–96.

Mayer, Emeran. *The Mind-Gut Connection: How the Hidden Conversation within Our Bodies Impacts Our Mood, Our Choices, and Our Overall Health*. New York: Harper Wave, 2018. Kindle.

McCullough, David. *The Great Bridge: The Epic Story of the Building of the Brooklyn Bridge*. New York: Simon & Schuster, 2012. Kindle.

Melfi, Theodore, dir. *Hidden Figures*. 2017; Beverly Hills, CA: Twentieth Century Fox Home Entertainment, 2017.

Merrell-Wolff, Franklin. *Pathways through to Space: A Personal Record of Transformation in Consciousness*. New York: Julian Press, 1973.

Miller, Suzy. *Awesomism! A New Way to Understand the Diagnosis of Autism*. n.p.: iUniverse, 2008.

Miller, Suzy, C. Reed, F. Tang, N. J. Manek, and W. A. Tiller WA. *Impact of Broadcast Intention on Autism Spectrum Behaviors*. In *International Research Congress on Integrative Medicine and Health (IRCIMH)*. Miami, FL: IRCIMH, 2014.

"MIT Team Achieves Coldest Temperature Ever." *MIT News*, September 11, 2003. Accessed January 16, 2019. http://news.mit.edu/2003/cooling.

Morowitz, Harold J. *Energy Flow in Biology*. Woodbridge, CT: Ox Bow Press, 1979.

Morowitz, Harold J. *Entropy for Biologists: An Introduction to Thermodynamics*. New York: Academic Press, 1973.

Morowitz, Harold J. *Mayonnaise and the Origin of Life: Thoughts of Minds and Molecules*. Woodbridge, CT: Ox Bow Press, 1991.

Murthy, Vivek. "Work and the Loneliness Epidemic: Reducing Isolation at Work Is Good for Business." *Harvard Business Review*, 2017. Accessed January 15, 2019. https://hbr.org/cover-story/2017/09/work-and-the-loneliness-epidemic.

Nasruddin. "The Lamp and the Key." The Outrageous Wisdom of Nasruddin. Accessed May 22, 2019. www.nasruddin.org/pages/storylist.html#lampandkey.

National Institutes for Health. "The BRAIN Initiative." Accessed March 15, 2019. www.braininitiative.nih.gov/.

National Institutes for Health. "The NIH Blueprint for Neuroscience Research." Accessed March 15, 2019. https://neuroscienceblueprint.nih.gov/.

National Institute of Environmental Health Sciences. "High Impact Journals: Superfund Research Program." NIEHS website.

Accessed January 24, 2019. https://tools.niehs.nih.gov/srp/publications/highimpactjournals.cfm.

Neff, Kristin D. "The Development and Validation of a Scale to Measure Self-Compassion." *Self and Identity* 2, no. 3 (2003): 223–50.

Niemtzow, R. C. "Acupuncture and Magnets: Is There a Clinical Role?" *Medical Acupuncture* 29, no. 5 (2017): 255–56.

Nobel Media. *The Nobel Prize in Chemistry 1977.* Accessed April 12, 2019. www.nobelprize.org/prizes/chemistry/1977/summary/.

Nobel Media. *The Nobel Prize in Physics 1978.* Accessed January 21, 2019. www.nobelprize.org/prizes/physics/1978/summary/.

Nørretranders, Tor. *The User Illusion: Cutting Consciousness Down to Size.* London: Penguin, 1999.

Nori, Franco. "Statistical Mechanics and Thermodynamics." Physics 406, Fall 1998. Accessed March 14, 2019. www-personal.umich.edu/~nori/course/physics_406_quotes.html.

Oschman, James L. *Energy Medicine in Therapeutics and Human Performance.* Edinburgh: Butterworth-Heinemann, 2003.

Pajunen, Grazyna A., Marguerite J. Purnell, Walter E. Dibble Jr., and William A. Tiller. "Altering the Acid/Alkaline Balance of Water via the Use of an Intention-Host Device." *Journal of Alternative and Complementary Medicine* 15, no. 9 (2009): 963–68.

Patten, Leslie, and Terry Patten. *Biocircuits: Amazing New Tools for Energy Health.* Tiburon, CA: H. J. Kramer, 1989.

Peterson, Jordan B. *12 Rules for Life: An Antidote to Chaos.* Toronto: Random House Canada, 2018. Kindle.

Perrin, Jean. *Atoms,* translated by D. L. Hammick. Woodbridge, CT: Ox Bow Press, 1990.

Pressfield, Steven. *Turning Pro: Tap Your Inner Power and Create Your Life's Work*. New York: Black Irish Entertainment, 2012. Kindle.

Pressfield, Steven. *The War of Art: Break through the Blocks and Win Your Inner Creative Battles*. New York: Black Irish Entertainment, 2012. Kindle.

Repcheck, Jack. *Copernicus' Secret: How the Scientific Revolution Began*. New York: Simon & Schuster, 2007. Kindle.

Robins, Richard W., Holly M. Hendin, and Kali H. Trzesniewski. "Measuring Global Self-Esteem: Construct Validation of a Single-Item Measure and the Rosenberg Self-Esteem Scale." *Personality and Social Psychology Bulletin* 27, no. 2 (2001): 151–61.

Rodis-Lewis, Genevieve. *Descartes: His Life and Thought*. Ithaca, NY: Cornell University Press. 1999.

Rosch, Paul J. *Bioelectromagnetic and Subtle Energy Medicine*. 2nd ed. Boca Raton, FL: CRC Press, 2015.

Rosenbaum, Lisa. "Resisting the Suppression of Science." *New England Journal of Medicine* 376, no. 17 (2017): 1607–609.

Rovelli, Carlo. *The Order of Time,* translated by Erica Segre and Simon Carnell. New York: Penguin, 2018. Kindle.

Rustum, Roy, William A. Tiller, Iris Bell, and M. Richard Hoover. "The Structure of Liquid Water; Novel Insights from Materials Research; Potential Relevance to Homeopathy." *Materials Research Innovations* 9, no. 4 (2005): 98–103.

Saydah, S. H., and M. S. Eberhardt. "Use of Complementary and Alternative Medicine among Adults with Chronic Diseases: United States 2002." *Journal of Alternative and Complementary Medicine* 12, no. 8 (2006): 805–812.

Schilpp, Paul Arthur et al. *The Library of Living Philosophers.*

Edited by P. A. Schilpp. Evanston, IL: Northwestern University, 1939.

Schrödinger, Erwin. *What Is Life?* Cambridge: Cambridge University Press, 2017.

Schumacher, E. F. *A Guide for the Perplexed.* Reissued edition. New York: Harper Perennial, 2015.

Schwartz, Stephan A. "Finding Saddam Hussein: A Study in Applied Remote Viewing." *EdgeScience,* 2018. Accessed April 23, 2019. www.scientificexploration.org/edgescience.

Shachtman, Tom. "The Coldest Place in the Universe." *Smithsonian Magazine,* January 2008. Accessed April 3, 2019. www.smithsonianmag.com/science-nature/the-coldest-place-in-the-universe-8121922.

Shannon, C. E. "A Mathematical Theory of Communication." *The Bell System Technical Journal* 27, no. 3 (1948): 379–423.

Shorto, Russel. *Descartes' Bones: A Skeletal History of the Conflict between Faith and Reason.* New York: Doubleday, 2008. Kindle.

Smith, C. W. "CAM in Camera." *Journal of Alternative and Complementary Medicine* 13, no. 1 (2007): 3–4.

Snow, C. P. *The Two Cultures and the Scientific Revolution.* Mansfield Center, CT: Martino, 2013.

Sobel, Dava. *A More Perfect Heaven: How Copernicus Revolutionized the Cosmos.* London: Bloomsbury, 2012. Kindle.

Soni, Jimmy, and Rob Goodman. *A Mind at Play: How Claude Shannon Invented the Information Age.* New York: Simon & Schuster, 2018. Kindle.

Stanford Encyclopedia of Philosophy. "René Descartes." Published December 3, 2009, revised January 16, 2014. Accessed March 12, 2019. https://plato.stanford.edu/entries/descartes/.

Stern, Joanna. "We Were Promised Mind-Blowing Personal Tech. What's the Hold-Up?" *Wall Street Journal,* May 3, 2018. Accessed March 12, 2019. www.wsj.com/articles/we-were-promised-mind-blowing-personal-tech-whats-the-hold-up-1525356604.

Stewart, Ian. *Why Beauty Is Truth: The History of Symmetry.* New York: Basic Books, 2008.

Strong, Mary. *Letters of the Scattered Brotherhood.* San Francisco: Harper and Row, 1991.

Sutton, Christine. "Hidden Symmetry: The Yang–Mills Equation." In *It Must Be Beautiful: Great Equations of Modern Science,* edited by Graham Farmelo, 231–52 London: Granta, 2003.

't Hooft, Gerard. "Gauge Theories of the Forces between Elementary Particles." *Scientific American* 242, no. 6 (June 1980): 104–41.

Targ, Russel, and Harold E. Puthoff. *Mind-Reach: Scientists Look at Psychic Abilities.* Charlottesville, VA: Hampton Roads, 2005.

Taylor, John. *Superminds: An Investigation into the Paranormal.* London: Picador, 1976.

Teller, Astro. *Astro Teller Captain Moonshots,* in *The Tim Ferriss Show.* 2018, Tim Ferriss San Francisco. Accessed January 15, 2019. www.youtube.com/watch?v=-gJAwCtqaWg.

Thakar, Vimala. *Insights into the Bhagavad Gita.* Delhi: Motilal Banarsidass, 2005.

Thomas, Lewis. *Lives of a Cell: Notes of a Biology Watcher.* New York: Penguin, 1982. Kindle.

Thomas, Lewis. *The Medusa and the Snail: More Notes of a Biology Watcher.* New York: Penguin, 1995. Kindle.

Tiller, William A. "A Gas Discharge Device for Investigating Focused Human Attention." *Journal of Scientific Exploration* 4, no. 2

(1990): 255–71.

Tiller, William A. "Electromagnetism versus Bioelectromagnetism." *Bioelectromagnetic and Subtle Energy Medicine,* 2nd edn. Edited by P. J. Rosch, 57–63. 2015. Kindle.

Tiller, William A. *Lectures on Psychoenergetic Science: A Second Copernican-Scale Revolution.* Directed by Ana Sanjuan. Denver, CO: University of Denver: Five DVD set, 2007.

Tiller, William A. *Psychoenergetic Science: A Second Copernican-Scale Revolution.* Walnut Creek, CA: Pavior, 2007.

Tiller, William A. "The Real World of Modern Science, Medicine, and Qigong." *Bulletin of Science, Technology and Society* 22, no. 5 (2002): 352–61.

Tiller, William A. *Science and Human Transformation: Subtle Energies, Intentionality, and Consciousness.* Walnut Creek, CA: Pavior, 1997.

Tiller, William A. "Towards a Predictive Model of Subtle Domain Connections to the Physical Domain Aspect of Reality: The Origins of Wave-Particle Duality, Electric-Magnetic Monopoles and the Mirror Principle." *Journal of Scientific Exploration* 13, no. 1 (1999): 41–67.

Tiller, William A. "What Are Subtle Energies?" *Journal of Scientific Exploration* 7, no. 3 (1993): 293–304.

Tiller, William A. *White Paper XV: Preventive Medicine/Self-Healing via One's Personal Biofield Pumping and Balancing.* Payson, AZ: William A. Tiller Institute, n.d.

Tiller, William A., and W. E. Dibble. *White Paper I: A Brief Introduction to Intention-Host Device Research,* n.d., accessed March 15, 2019. www.tiller.org.

Tiller, William A., and Walter E. Dibble Jr. *Conscious Acts of*

Creation: The Emergence of a New Physics. Walnut Creek, CA: Pavior, 2001.

Tiller, William A., and Walter E. Dibble Jr. "Expanding Thermodynamic Perspective for Materials in SU (2) Electromagnetic (EM) Gauge Symmetry State Space: Part 1, Duplex Space Model with Applications to Homeopathy." *Materials Research Innovations* 11, no. 4 (2007): 163–68.

Tiller, William, and Walter E. Dibble Jr. "Expanding Thermodynamic Perspective for Materials in SU (2) EM Gauge Symmetry State Space: Part 2–Magnetoelectrochemical Potential Energy Detector." *Materials Research Innovations* 12, no. 3 (2008): 107–13.

Tiller, William A., and Walter E. Dibble Jr. "New Experimental Data Revealing an Unexpected Dimension to Materials Science and Engineering." *Materials Research Innovations* 5, no. 1 (2001): 21–34.

Tiller, William A., and Walter E. Dibble Jr. "Toward General Experimentation and Discovery in Conditioned Laboratory and Complementary and Alternative Medicine Spaces: Part V. Data on 10 Different Sites Using a Robust New Type of Subtle Energy Detector." *Journal of Alternative and Complementary Medicine* 13, no. 1 (2007): 133–49.

Tiller, William A., Walter E. Dibble, and Michael J. Kohane. "Towards Objectifying Intention via Electronic Devices." *Subtle Energies and Energy Medicine* 8, no. 2 (1999): 103–23.

Tiller, William A., Walter E. Dibble, G. Orlando, A. Migli, G. Raiteri, and J. Oca. "Toward General Experimentation and Discovery in Conditioned Laboratory Spaces: Part IV. Macroscopic Information Entanglement between Sites Approximately 6000

Miles Apart." *Journal of Alternative and Complementary Medicine* 11, no. 6 (2005): 973–76.

Tiller, William A., Elmer E. Green, Peter A. Parks, and Stacy Anderson. "Towards Explaining Anomalously Large Body Voltage Surges on Exceptional Subjects Part I: The Electrostatic Approximation." *Journal of Scientific Exploration* 9, no. 3 (1995): 331–50.

Tiller, William A., Michael J. Kohane, and Walter E. Dibble. "Can an Aspect of Consciousness Be Imprinted into an Electronic Device?" *Integrative Physiological and Behavioral Science* 35, no. 2 (2000): 142–62.

Tiller, William A., S. Miller, C. R. Reed, F. Tang, N. Manek, and W. E. Dibble Jr. *White Paper XXXI. The Globally Broadcast Autism Intention Experiment: Part II. Some ATEC Trends and Statistical Data for a Twelve-Month Program.* Payson, AZ: Tiller Institute, 2014.

Tiller, William A., S. Miller, C. R. Reed, and J. Yotopoulos. *White Paper XXX. The Globally Broadcast Autism Intention Experiment: Part I, at the Four-Month Stage of a Twelve-Month Program.* Payson, AZ: Tiller Institute, 2013.

Tiller, William A., Jean E. Tiller, Walter E. Dibble, Raj Manek, and Nisha J. Manek. "The Buddha Relics and Evidence of Physical Space Conditioning with Unimprinted Intention Host Devices." *Journal of Alternative and Complementary Medicine* 18, no. 4 (2012): 379–81.

Uys, Jamie, dir. *The Gods Must Be Crazy.* 2004; Culver City, CA: Columbia TriStar Home Entertainment, 1980.

Van Ness, H. C., *Understanding Thermodynamics.* New York: McGraw-Hill, 1969. Kindle.

Vedral, Vlatko. *Decoding Reality: The Universe as Quantum Information.* Oxford: Oxford University Press, 2018. Kindle.

Wagner, Erica. *Chief Engineer: Washington Roebling, the Man Who Built the Brooklyn Bridge.* New York: Bloomsbury, 2017. Kindle.

Waldrop, M. Mitchell. "Claude Shannon: Reluctant Father of the Digital Age." *MIT Technology Review,* July 1, 2001. Accessed April 3, 2019. www.technologyreview.com/s/401112/claude-shannon-reluctant-father-of-the-digital-age/.

Wang, Chenchen, Christopher H. Schmid, Ramel Bones, Robert Kalish, Janeth Yinh, Don L. Goldenberg, Yoojin Yee, and Timothy McAlindon. "A Randomized Trial of Tai Chi for Fibromyalgia." *New England Journal of Medicine* 363, no. 8 (2010): 743–54.

Watson, Lyall. *Gifts of Unknown Things: A True Story of Nature, Healing, and Initiation from Indonesia's "Dancing Island."* Rochester, VT: Destiny Books, 1991.

Watson, Lyall. *The Nature of Things: The Secret Life of Inanimate Objects.* Rochester, VT: Destiny Books, 1992.

The Weather Channel. "Polar Vortex Triggers Coldest Arctic Outbreak in at Least Two Decades in Parts of the Midwest." January 31, 2019. https://weather.com/forecast/national/news/2019-01-28-polar-vortex-midwest-arctic-air-coldest-two-decades.

West, C. P., L. N. Dyrbye, and T. D. Shanafelt. "Physician Burnout: Contributors, Consequences and Solutions." *Journal of Internal Medicine* 283, no. 6 (2018): 516–29.

Weyl, Hermann. *Symmetry.* Princeton Science Library reprint edition. Princeton, NJ: Princeton University Press, 2016.

Wikipedia. "John G. Taylor." Accessed March 16, 2019. https://

en.wikipedia.org/wiki/John_G._Taylor.

Wikipedia. "Self-Ionization of Water." Accessed April 23, 2019. https://en.wikipedia.org/wiki/Self-ionization_of_water.

Wilczek, Frank. "A Piece of Magic: The Dirac Equation." *It Must Be Beautiful: Great Equations of Modern Science*. Edited by Graham Farmelo, 132–60. London: Granta, 2003.

Wolchover, N. "A New Physics Theory of Life." *Quanta Magazine*. January 22, 2014. www.quantamagazine.org/a-new-thermodynamics-theory-of-the-origin-of-life-20140122/

Yam, Philip. "Exploiting Zero-Point Energy." *Scientific American* 277, no. 6 (1997): 82–85.

Yeung, A. W., T. K. Goto, and W. K. Leung. "The Changing Landscape of Neuroscience Research, 2006-2015: A Bibliometric Study." *Frontiers in Neuroscience* 11 (2017): 120.

Yogananda, Paramhansa. *Autobiography of a Yogi*. Los Angeles: Self-Realization Fellowship, 2017. Kindle.

Zimmerman, M. "Neurophysiology of Sensory Systems." *Fundamentals of Sensory Physiology*. Edited by Robert F. Schmidt, 68–116. Berlin: Springer, 1986.

INDEX

ILLUSTRATION CREDITS

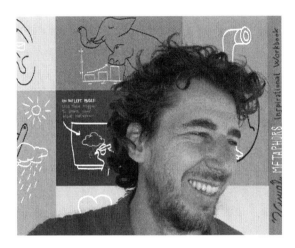

Dario Paniagua hails from Buenos Aires, Argentina, and worked in the advertising industry at Young & Rubicam and Saatchi and Saatchi before transitioning to what he truly loves: teaching people to discover their hidden artistic abilities. To keep his imagination nimble, Dario watches cartoons, builds with LEGOs, plays board games, and continually creates new information by drawing and doodling. He has authored two books, *Visual Speaking Like a Boss* and *Visual Metaphors Inspirational Workbook.* Since 2003, he has lived in Lecco, Italy, and gives workshops all over the world. Visit him online at: **https://dariopaniagua.com.**

Nisha's first lesson in thermodynamics, written by Dr. Tiller

$$\underline{THERMO}$$

$U(1)\ GAUGE\ (D\text{-}SPACE\text{-}ONLY\ )$

ELECTROCHEMICAL POTENTIAL

CONCENTRATION

$$G = pV + F - TS = \sum_j \eta_j\ c_j$$

D-SPACE

THE j^{TH} SPECIES

$$\eta_j = \mu_j + z_j e\phi + \dots$$

CHEMICAL POTENTIAL

$z =$ VALENCE

$e =$ ELECTON CHARGE

$\phi =$ ELECTRICAL POTENTIAL (VOLTAGE)

$$\mu_j = \mu_{0j} + k_B T \ln_e a_j$$

CHEMICAL ACTIVITY $= \gamma_j c_j$

THERMODYNAMIC ACTIVITY COEFFICIENT

$\Delta G > 0 \rightarrow$ WORK

MIX OF $SU(2)$ & $U(1)$

$$G_{D/R} = V_{SU(2)}\ G_{SU(2)} + (1 - V_{SU(2)})\ G_D \quad // \quad \alpha_{eff} \propto \frac{V_{SU(2)}}{V_{U(1)}}$$

$V_{U(1)}$

ABOUT THE AUTHOR

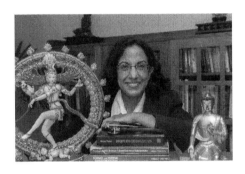

Nisha J. Manek was born on the equator in the village of Ol'Kalou in Nyahururu district in the highlands of Kenya. She graduated *summa cum laude* from Case Western Reserve University in Cleveland, Ohio, after which she received her doctorate in medicine with commendation from Glasgow University School of Medicine, Glasgow, Scotland. She completed her fellowship in rheumatology at Stanford University Medical Center, Palo Alto, California, and joined the faculty as Assistant Professor of Medicine at the Mayo Clinic, Rochester, Minnesota. She has served on many academic committees, including the Association of Rheumatology Health Professionals (ARHP) of the American College of Rheumatology. She is an invited faculty member for the associate fellowship program in integrative medicine at the University of Arizona, Tucson. In this capacity, she writes the integrative rheumatology curriculum. Dr. Manek has authored more than a dozen book chapters for academic medical textbooks. She is a fellow of the American College of Physicians and a Fellow of the Royal College of Physicians (Glasgow) of the United Kingdom. She is usually busy creating new "information" in her clinic.

Visit her at: **www.NishaManekMD.com** and pick up your copy of the scientific paper on the sacred Buddha relics.

Manufactured by Amazon.ca
Bolton, ON